The
Medical Handbook
to end all
Medical Handbooks

The
Medical Handbook
to end all
Medical Handbooks

Dr. L. PHEASANT

Illustrations by Paul Rigby

WOLFE PUBLISHING LIMITED

First published 1974 by
Wolfe Publishing Limited
10 Earlham Street
London WC2H 9LP

Copyright © Dr. L. Pheasant 1974

SBN 7234 0538 7

Printed by The Garden City Press Limited
Letchworth, Hertfordshire SG6 1JS

Contents

Contents

Children under the age of eighteen years are advised not to read this book unless accompanied by an adult.

Introduction

OVER countless years there have been countless numbers of medical handbooks. I hope this will be the last.

L.P.

CHAPTER ONE

Doctors

DOCTORING is one of the strangest professions ever. Most people who have never been doctors, after their twelfth pint of beer or fifth gin, will confide that, although they have made five million pounds selling fancy hats for carnivals, all they have ever really wanted to be is a doctor. They can remember, at the age of three, their Aunty Fanny saying they had surgeon's hands when they had de-winkled a winkle shell without a pin. Doctors, on the other hand, as soon as they become doctors, always want to be something else. So you have farming doctors, fishing doctors, politician doctors, dancing doctors, climbing doctors, flying doctors, swimming doctors, journalist doctors, mining doctors, radio and television doctors and, of course, Naval, Army and Air Force doctors, all of whom say how helpful their medical knowledge is in their new career. Be reassured, at the last count, there were still three doctoring doctors working in the British Isles alone.

There are brown doctors, white doctors, yellow doctors, pink doctors, alcoholic doctors, and a few rare mauve doctors.

Alcoholic doctors are always liked the best because (a) they are so obviously sensible in staying drunk all the time, and (b) the patients will say 'I know he's one for the booze, but he's marvellous when he's sober'.

There are one-armed doctors, one-legged doctors, one-eyed doctors, bald doctors, hairy doctors, shaggy doctors, one-eared doctors, no-eared doctors, thin doctors, fat doctors, short doctors, tall doctors, tiny doctors, midget doctors, sexy doctors, frigid doctors, warm doctors, kind doctors, unkind doctors, polite doctors, rude doctors, grumpy doctors, smiling doctors, frowning doctors, winking doctors, spitting doctors, smoking doctors, frying doctors (I must check this), lady doctors, men doctors, boy doctors, girl doctors, old lady doctors, old men doctors, middle aged doctors, non-smoking doctors, drug taking doctors, mad doctors, senile doctors, toothless doctors, doctors with false teeth, doctors with gold teeth, atomic doctors, steam doctors (I must check this), coal doctors, tree doctors, holiday camp doctors, hotel doctors, airport doctors, night club doctors, football doctors, boxing doctors, librarian doctors, engineering doctors, society doctors, working class doctors, middle class doctors, conservative doctors, liberal doctors, anarchist doctors, Muslim doctors, Hindu doctors, British doctors, Presbyterian doctors, Roman Catholic doctors, Church of England doctors, Methodist doctors, witch doctors, village doctors, town doctors, city doctors.

This covers, broadly, the range of normal doctors. Then there are the other doctors who, as well as practising medicine, have to cope with some personal affliction of their own. There are knock-kneed doctors, pigeon-toed doctors, doctors with facial ticks, and cross-eyed doctors. I am particularly conscious of the troubles of this group, as it is in this category that I place myself.

Afflictions and disabilities, like beauty, are only skin deep, but whereas you could probably live quite happily with a man who had lost a leg, it is almost certain that you would be unable to tolerate life with someone who ate peas off a knife.

Appearance Alcoholic

The less the apparent significance of an affliction or disability, the more sinister are its aspects, and I suffer from one of the most insidious of all—I look like a whisky drinker.

Apart from an occasional sherry and the odd glass of wine with a meal, alcohol on the whole is distasteful to me, but cruel nature has so shaped my features that anyone, whether known

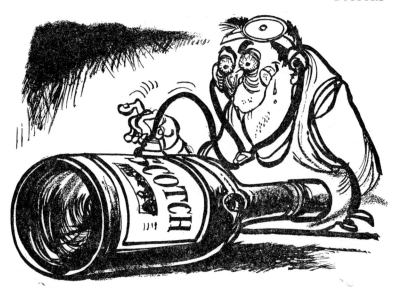

to me or not, as soon as he sees me, is seized with an impulse to
rush off and fetch me a glass of whisky.

This would not at first appear to be too great a handicap. But
I can go to a sherry or cheese and wine party in a house that is
completely strange to me, and an unknown and unmet host will
be pouring out drinks. Having attended to the rest of whichever
party I am with, will either say (in spite of my protests) 'I am
sure you would rather have a whisky' or just shove a tumbler
full of the neat stuff into my hand, while I cast envious eyes
round at the rest of the company who are enjoying the proferred
sherry or wine, which is the only refreshment I really like.

It has begun to handicap my work. Night calls have become
extremely dangerous. Without exception, in households that can
afford to keep a liquor stock, at the end of my nocturnal
examination, a half to one tumbler full of whisky is thrust into
my hand as I come down the stairs, making it impossible to get
my coat on till I have drunk it. If I try to refuse it they think I
have been offended by the lateness of the call.

The speed at which I drink it, in order to get away, confirms
their belief about my addiction and their thoughts that, without
a stiff peg, I wouldn't even reach my car.

If I happen to get called out twice in the same night, I go to the second call already smelling of whisky, which eliminates any chance of getting away without a further dose.

I have lived long enough in the same place now to have begun to suffer the side effects of my affliction. Anybody who feels that I have in some small way helped him, knows that he can always reward me by giving me a bottle of whisky. There are bottles left in the surgery, either with notes or anonymously. Bottles are thrust into my hand as I leave households. They are even left surreptitiously on my car seat, always with the same message— 'To be saved until you get home'. At Christmas it arrives by the van load, and I have now built up one of the largest stocks of whisky in the district.

Purely to economize on room, on the slightest pretext, I give away as much as I possibly can. This only heightens the impression that in my household whisky flows more readily than water, and that water doesn't mix with it anyway.

Every Budget Day I pray that the Chancellor will have mercy on me and double the tax on this commodity. The abolition of resale price maintenance is as big a blow to me personally as the retreat from Dunkirk.

In spite of whatever idiosyncrasies a doctor may have or suffer from, he must still practise this work of medicine, though that idiosyncrasy may dominate the way he practises it.

Thus, doctors practise their medicine in different ways.

Some are outward-going, jolly fellows, jovial, well-met types; some are deaf, some are dreary, some are shy, and some are aggressive and rude.

Most don't like to be contradicted and, if you should be foolish enough to self-diagnose or self-prescribe in front of them, even if you are right, you can bet your bottom dollar you will finish up with neither your diagnosis nor your treatment. Some are friendly and do their best for you; others are spiteful, and will put a laxative, unbeknown to you, in your medicine just to keep you down a peg.

Doctors have to appear all-wise and all-knowing, and have an answer for all questions even if, as it often happens, they don't know anything and give the wrong answers. The only time in my own particular experience when I have been unable to give a 'yes' or 'no' answer was when a woman patient rang me in the middle of a busy surgery to tell me that her son had won a piano playing competition—should he cut a record for the first time ever? I had to say I didn't know.

Doctor's Problems

Patients get attached to their doctors, and send them presents at Christmas. This is quite selfless, though in identifying themselves when asking for a home visit the patient says, 'I'm Mrs. Jenkins who sent your children some sweets at Christmas'. It is important also for the doctor to remember to wear the right hand-knitted socks when going to the right patient, and when a patient brings a large bottle to the house not to thank the giver too effusively until he has discovered whether it is gin or urine.

These are some of the many problems the doctor has.

Take, for example, the newly qualified doctor strolling into a pub in the heart of his new practice. He is eyed suspiciously at first by the dominoes and darts players, and then ignored until he approaches the bar. The following conversation ensues:

Doctor: 'A pint of bitter, please.'

Landlord (conducting a brief non-medical examination while pulling a pint): Stranger here, sir?'

Doctor: 'That's right. I've just moved to this area.'

Landlord: 'Work bring you here sir?'

Doctor: 'Right again.'

Brief silence ensues until the doctor feels compelled to qualify his reply.

'Well, actually, I'm the new doctor.'

At this point the lights in the pub, previously dimmed, suddenly sparkle at full wattage. Chairs are pushed aside, drinks are spilled, rows of dominoes topple, and darts fall unheeded into pints of light and mild. In about three seconds our young doctor finds a queue of locals in front of him, asking questions about hernias, piles, game legs, the effect of gin and orange on sexual potency, whether dogs can have venereal disease, and the invariable claims: 'You must come and have a look at our

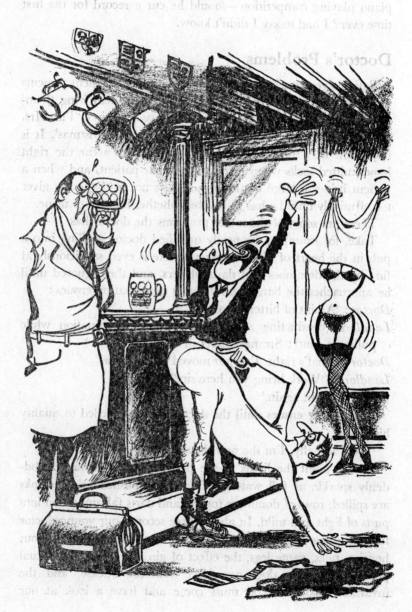

Dennis, Doc; they say he's got the biggest !! this side of Bridlington'.

This is only the beginning of his troubles.

Pursued by Sex

If the doctor is young and single, young and married, or any one of these combinations through middle-age and old-age, sex will pursue him throughout his career.

Many a young doctor has glanced at the appointment list for his coming surgery and has only saved his life and professional reputation by leaping into a cold bath and soaking for ten minutes before seeing the first patient.

The prospect of examining fifteen marriageable ladies, all for sale, and armed with black suspender belts, during the course of the morning has been the reason for many a young doctor joining the Foreign Legion.

The popularity of women's tights has greatly relieved the tension in this area as these are the most sexless piece of wearing apparel ever invented. However smart or beautifully dressed the woman patient may be, by the time she has rolled her tights down below her knees and waddled across the consulting room like a refugee from a chain gang, whatever slim chance of seduction she had has gone.

As one 15-stone patient related to me, discussing women's wearing apparel nowadays, he had watched his 15-stone wife kit herself up for the day—she put on pants, belt, tights, long woollen drawers, slacks, then preened herself in the mirror. 'Well,' said my 15-stone friend, 'if anyone rapes you to-day, he deserves to get away with it.'

There have always been doctors; there will always be doctors. They are a mixture of magic, medicine and make-believe. If you cannot do with them, you cannot do without them.

CHAPTER TWO

Nurses

THERE ARE fat nurses, thin nurses, efficient nurses, sexy nurses, male and female nurses. Like doctors, they are of every creed and colour but, unlike doctors, they are all quite lovely.

Shapely Angels

They are the best part of any medical service. Cool, comforting, delicious angels, the rounded contours of their starched upper aprons being the main factors in reviving male patients and giving them something to live for. Up until the most recent designs, nurses' uniforms gave them a mystique, an aura of mystery. How much of their shape was starch, and how much woman, and how to find out. The full bosomed, starched and bonneted angel at your bedside can, as a date for the pictures, turn out to be anything from a double of Sophia Loren to a flat-chested girl in an ill-fitting tweed suit with holes in her stockings. You pays yer money and you gets no choice.

To be a good nurse you have to have a vocation; in fact all nurses have a vocation, so by definition, should be good. The vocation is not to comfort the sick and injured, it's simply to find a doctor for a husband. As there are not enough doctors to go round, many will have to lower their sights and marry men like solicitors, policemen, and newspaper editors.

There are very few doctors who are not married to nurses, and the few doctors who do marry non-nurses tend to get bald and fat at a very premature age.

Nurses, once they have decided they are not going to get a doctor husband, have unique opportunities for selecting a mate as, before they even speak to a potential husband, they have a good chance of rubbing him down and assessing his basic essentials, whereas the poor non-nurse wife may not (but not so commonly in this day and age) find out most of the horrible truths about her partner until the actual wedding night. Not only has the nurse seen and assessed before talking, but also has opportunities for further assessment when in doubt by actually taking measurements with compasses and contractors next time her 'possible' has an anaesthetic.

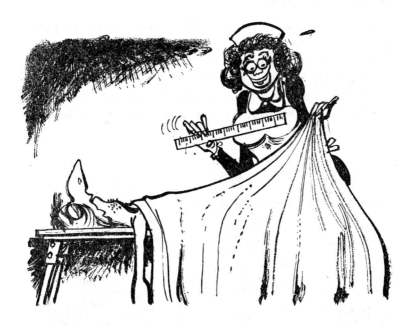

Apart from the different shapes, colours, and sizes of nurses, there are, in fact, many different types of nurse. There are:

Student nurses	Midwives	District nurses
Children's nurses	Industrial nurses	
Ward nurses	School Matrons	

and, not the least, **Male nurses**.

When a sergeant-major status is reached in the nursing profession, you are given the title 'Sister', even if you haven't got a moustache. Even ranking male nurses are called 'Sister'—it's enough to drive anyone gay. There are:

Outpatients' sisters	Theatre sisters, and
Ward sisters	Night sisters.

Whatever named branch of medicine, there is a sister for it. Thus, there are plastic sisters (many), chest sisters, orthopaedic sisters, surgical sisters, E.N.T. sisters, and so on.

Student Nurses

Student nurses are nurses under scrutiny, who are in the process of deciding whether they really want to be nurses, while they are watched by hawk-eyed, fiery sisters, who decide if they have the stuff in them to make the grade. It was a student nurse who didn't make the grade who was admonished by Sister when the Sister heard screams, and saw steam coming from behind a

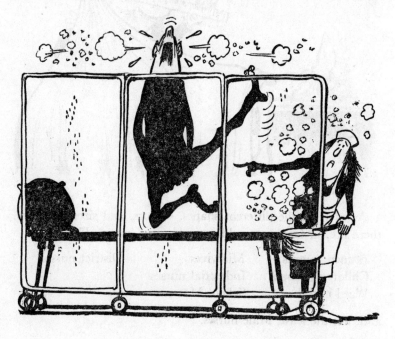

screen in the men's surgical ward. 'No, no, nurse,' the Sister shouted, 'I told you to prick his boil.'

It was another non-grader of this type who, in an examination, defined hard water as 'ice', and the way to soften it, 'to melt it'. She could be right.

Student nurses carry out all the most menial tasks, like washing bed pans, emptying urinals, and in this particular situation, when one is described as 'a good little scrubber', it is no reflection on how she dispenses her female favours but an appreciation of her ability to make the latrine floor shine.

If she survives these first three months, the student nurse is given a different uniform, and starts either a two-year course as a State Enrolled Nurse or a three-year course as a State Registered Nurse.

During these years they have a confusing system of coloured belts to show how well (or badly) they are getting on. If, eventually, they survive their training, they are then able to aim for higher posts, such as Staff Nurse, Sister, Matron, etc.

Children's Nurses

Children's nurses are an undefined group, varying from voluptuous Swedish au pair girls to highly qualified paediatric nurses. Many of these dolly Swedes, as described, have no idea when answering advertisements that they are going to be the actual mother of the children.

This branch of nursing is popular, as you can start training earlier than in other branches. It is excellent training for

1. Coping with children you are likely to have yourself in years to come
2. Coping with lecherous middle-aged fathers trying to regain their youth.

Ward Nurses

Ward nurses are nurses who have passed the probationer stage and are let loose on the ward for two or three years' training. They have to learn all the practical procedures—blanket bathing, dressings, bandaging, how to give injections, put up transfusions, and give enemas.

It was a cross-eyed nurse who, on a week of enema duty, gave rise to three complaints and five excited commendations from lady patients. She was subsequently ordered to get new glasses, and sent back to the training range.

Night Duty Infirmary

During these years the nurse has her best chance of getting her doctor husband—intimate cups of coffee on night duty, boozy hospital dances, and uncomfortable hours on touchlines supporting Rugby teams. If the nurse is at a teaching hospital she will have the added bonus/disadvantage of medical students, who require a book of their own.

They highly increase the prospect of medical marriage, but also highly increase the chance that the embryo doctor will be using the nurse only to brush up on his anatomy.

District Nurses

District nurses do not work in hospitals but drive round the country in mini motorcars, nursing people at home. They are an integral part of the community, and know more domestic secrets than doctors. They are experts on constipation, blanket bathing, and varicose ulcers, and can always get their own back on people they don't like by giving them double influenza vaccinations in the buttock, stopping their enemies from sitting down comfortably for the next couple of weeks.

District nurses sometimes double as midwives and deliver babies at home. They know even more about the community secrets than ordinary district nurses, and are in great demand as judges for Baby Shows. Only once in my long experience as a general practitioner was I ever foolish enough to trespass in this territory.

Doctor's Dilemma

When you first qualify in medicine, you are warned of various pitfalls, such as becoming too familiar with patients of the opposite sex, or lending money, or advertising. The one great omission in this early briefing seems to be that no one warns unwary practitioners of the hazards of judging Baby Shows.

I accepted my first and only invitation to judge a Baby Show in an off guarded moment when I was leaving a house in a hurry. Full realisation did not fall upon me until two months later, at the Vicar's Garden Party, when I walked into a small tent next to a bulging marquee, to be confronted by six babies, each one with a supporting troupe of at least four relatives.

I like babies, and most of them are fit and thriving and I know no way of deciding whether one is any better than another. Seeing six in front of me being sat on the table, I thought my afternoon's work could be easily and methodically done.

I examined each baby carefully, making notes in my notebook for points that might help in my final decision. As I examined the second baby in the row, I realised it wasn't going to be easy at all. The mother smiled and said,

'Don't you remember, doctor, you delivered him last winter?' and looked knowingly as if to say, 'You are bound to pick one of your deliveries.'

I realised then, that if I picked a baby that I had delivered myself, or one of my partners' babies, there would be cries of 'favouritism'. If I didn't pick one belonging to our particular practice, the whole practice would probably leave us the next day.

It took me just over half an hour to make a complete examination. The lady organiser was fidgeting a bit. She said, with a nervous smile,

'There are quite a few more, doctor.'

A Glut Of Infants

I had thought it seemed too easy, and the bulging marquee next door I soon learnt contained flowing reinforcements to fill up the table in the smaller tent as soon as it had emptied.

'How many are there on the list altogether?' I asked.

'109, doctor, it's a record.'

I still had 103 to go!

Having spent so long on the first six, I could not really skimp the other 103. I did of course have to cut down my time. I battled on through the heat of the summer's afternoon, with two attendant reporters laboriously taking down the names and descriptions of each entrant. I had started at quarter to three, hoping to be finished by 4 p.m., but at 6.30, I had only reached number seventy-eight, and there was chaos in the supporting marquee.

Many of the entrants had not yet been weaned from the bottle and were having to be fed by the more portable supply of this type of food.

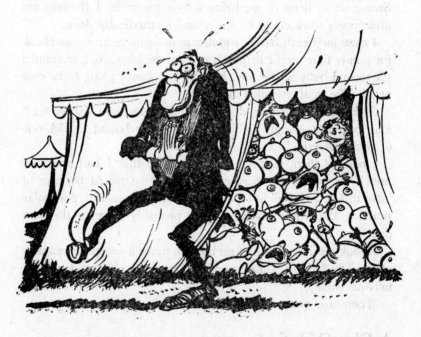

The bachelor curate, hearing the commotion that accompanies feeding time coming from the marquee, popped in, in his enthusiastic way, hoping to help and was met by a mass exhibition of breast feeding. He was led fainting away to the refreshment tent and given a glass of water.

I battled on, making copious notes, until at quarter past seven I had finished the last hundred and ninth.

Nobody had defaulted in the waiting time.

By my detailed system of elimination, which mainly consisted of babies with discharging ears and ones who had had bits bitten out of them by others whilst waiting to be exhibited, reduced my list down to seventy-five.

Twenty-four of these were attended by our own practice and fifty from practices round about, one single infant was staying on holiday. I picked a random twelve, including the holiday-maker, to be seen again. The weary mothers and screaming babies staggered back into the tent.

The reporters who had stuck loyally by me, recording through the whole ordeal, were in rebellion, grumbling in their beards,

'It's already two hours past opening time.'

In a fit of inspiration I decided on the only uncommitted child—the holidaymaker—as the winner, and staggered off to the refreshment tent.

The Vicar and the Organiser followed me quickly,

'I'm awfully sorry, doctor,' they said, 'the child should never have been entered, it doesn't fulfil the birthplace requisite in the entry form.'

I thumbed through my notes in despair. I couldn't honestly find any help to show that any one of the 109 babies was really any better than any other. They all looked jolly good specimens of budding male and femalehood to me.

I went back and scrutinised the remaining eleven finalists. I picked out six. Two that I had delivered, one that my partner had delivered, and one each from the other three practices in the town.

A Master Of Diplomacy

With some emotion and complete honesty, I got on to the rostrum and said,

'Ladies and Gentlemen. In all the Baby Shows that I have judged, I have never seen such a high standard of healthy, well brought up babies. It is impossible for me to name any single baby from amongst those entered. I therefore announce the following six all as winners, as they contained the eight points that I was looking for amongst the entrants. Bad luck to the losers, perhaps next time the judge will select different points on which to make his decision and it will be your turn to win.'

This was my last Baby Show ever. Some of my mothers and babies I had failed to select, transferred to other practices, and this was only to some extent compensated by the three finalists who weren't my patients transferring to me.

From then on I left this territory exclusively to the District Midwife.

Midwives

Midwives, as such, by and large, work only in hospitals. They become very dedicated to their work and amass great delivery scores like Test cricket heroes. No midwife ever scored a thousand before the end of May, but century scorers are two a penny, and, at midwives conventions, they sit and discuss the entries they have brought into the world. One midwife, listening to, and watching, a verbose politician on the television screen, commented, 'To think, if I hadn't originally slapped his bottom, he would never have uttered a word.'

Industrial Nurses

Industrial nurses are usually married, and spend most of their time in the Works' Canteen drinking tea, sending all accidents off to the nearest hospital. They are at their best when, on the firm's outing, they save many a life by knowing how to lay drunken workmates on their side (coma position) and remove their false teeth, thus largely reducing the danger of them drowning in the gallons of beer and cider they have just consumed.

They are worth employing for this duty alone.

School Matrons

School matrons have the unenviable task of not only looking after school children, but coping with their parents. There is no parent who doesn't think his child is the only child in the world. When you have 350 children to look after (boys or girls), and thus 700 parents to convince that you are just that bit more interested in the welfare of their Johnnie than any other child, there is nothing left to do but take to drink, jump in the river, or go to Singapore for Christmas.

Male Nurses

Male nursing, a most honourable profession, has yet to come fully into its own. Its peak will be reached when the mixed ward has become universally accepted. Until then, much of their activities will be confined to shaving old men who have water-works or pile trouble.

Sisters

Sisters are all-powerful, ruling the domain over which they preside with rods of iron.

Out Patient's Sisters

The toughest of the lot, usually experts in karate and judo, and when an obstreperous patient claims he was thrown out of the hospital, he is probably describing the overhead fling lock of the particular sister on duty.

Ward Sisters

Matriarchs whose administrative duties prevent them from doing practical nursing. Their main interests are straight bed covers, dust-free wards, and scaring the living daylights out of medical students and house surgeons.

Theatre Sisters

The sexiest of all nurses as they spend most of their day swathed, with only their eyes showing, and could get away with being mistaken for strict Muslims. They learn to speak with their eyes—a habit they cannot drop when they leave the theatre.

It is important to know the eye language since what you may translate as a covetous look from an attractive woman at a hospital dance, that encourages your prospects of a successful amorous evening, translated, probably means 'I know you, and don't you dare come into my theatre with suede shoes on again'.

Night Sisters

The real Florence Nightingales of the profession, flitting through the dark night, spreading comfort, sleeping in the daytime when all the world is about.

Do we ever realise how fortunate we are that women are prepared to give up their lives for nursing?

CHAPTER THREE

Medical Students

MEDICAL STUDENTS, of all students, have the undisputed claim to being the most irresponsible. There seems to be a set pattern in professional bodies that the more professional the body, the wilder the budding aspirants are during their training. There are few adventures and scrapes that general students have undergone that medical students have not perfected.

Medical students nominally spend five years at their medical school; the first two years studying anatomy and physiology, and the last three years walking the wards and studying clinical medicine.

Cutting Corners

There is a way of becoming a medical student before that, by spending a year cutting up dogfish and rabbits, making sections of plants and doing physics and chemistry, but this is generally part of the school curriculum.

It is this particular pre-medical group who are by far the most dangerous because, with the experience of having dissected one earth worm, a frog and two rabbits, they will venture to give a surgical opinion at any gathering, and are a hazard at a road accident or earthquake, because they will attempt with great courage any manipulation or straightening of bones from which their more experienced colleagues would flinch.

Happily, most of them do not get through their first-year

exam, the places being filled by schoolboys bristling with 'A'
Levels. Most settle down as publicans, always proud of the fact
that they were once medical students. They will be an authority
on all the local doctors, and will still give medical advice at the
drop of a hat.

The Good Old Days

Entrance to medical school is now all done by computers, and
much of the character has gone out of medical students and
medical schools.

When I was a medical student there was only one criterion for
admission to my hospital, and that was based on the ability to
play Rugby. Although the course was nominally five or six years,
there were several middle-aged gentlemen who had been happily
studying for fifteen or sixteen years, carrying on full-time jobs
such as chucker-outers in night clubs, hall porters, bookies'
runners, etc., to supplement their student's grant.

Skulduggery

It was my own prowess in Rugby that enabled me eventually
to qualify. Having failed several times, I approached the distinguished surgeon, President of our Rugby Club, explaining my
predicament, that I felt the time had really come for me to pass
and, knowing that he was on the Examination Board, asked if
there was any way he could help. Straight away he approached
his fellow examiners and said: 'Today, coming up for examination is our best Wing Three-Quarter. We cannot do without him
in the Rugby team; whatever you do, don't pass him.'

So his fellow examiners got together and said: 'Here's this
eminent surgeon, Sir Charlie Wrong, trying to prevent this
student, who is married with five children, from qualifying just
so that his own hospital will win the Hospital Cup. However he
does in the examination, we'll pass him.'

And this is how I came to qualify.

Dissecting the human body, which is half of the two-year
curriculum, brings one in contact with the harsh realities of life.
By the time you have spent two years chopping up your fellow

mortals in the company of a girl with a size 36 bust, 22 waist, 32 hips, you have few secrets from each other.

If you can say it was Miss Jones who helped you through your anatomy, you can bet she says it was you who helped her through hers, even if you did fumble a bit at first. Happily, since the appearance of the birth pill, there's a good chance of students qualifying without their unions being blessed.

Their Ill Spent Youth

Medical students, for some reason, are the most sexually active of all students, perhaps because they are so involved with the basic fundamentals of life during their years of study, they stick to basic fundamentals in their leisure time. When, in later life, you are paying substantial sums for cosmetic surgery and psycho-analysis sessions, little do you know that the two immaculately dressed gentlemen in striped shirts, with distant manners, used to be the famed Shagger Smith and Randy Robinson. The lack of community life after qualifying prevents access to the private lives of these remote gentlemen. It is probable that the flame flickers and dies a bit when the student becomes entitled to wear the magic name 'Doctor', but who knows the intimate secrets of some examination couches.

The Rugby Syndrome

Apart from sex, the main occupation of medical students is playing Rugby. Although they do play most other games as well, it is only Rugby that counts, and it is much more important that you should be picked to play for your Hospital First Fifteen than it is for you to pass your qualifying medical examinations. The association with Rugby never leaves the medical profession. When patients ask their G.P.'s for a specialist's opinion, they will not be referred to the best skin specialist in the land, or a surgeon who can take out a gall bladder with his eyes bandaged and one hand tied behind his back. It is much more likely that they will be told : 'I'll send you to see old Atkinson—he was the best fly-half we ever had', or 'I'll see if I can get an appointment with Perkins—he used to play on the wing for England'.

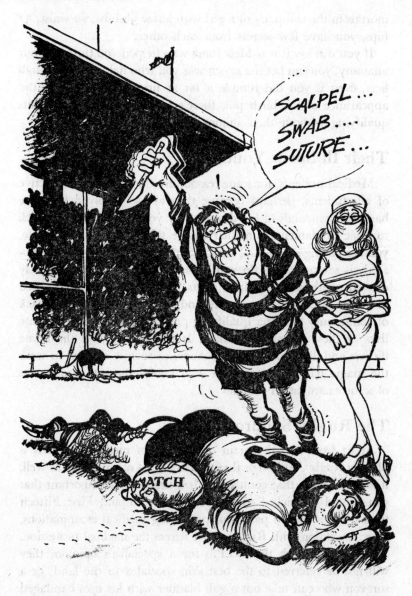

Rugby football does widen the horizons of medical students. As they spend so much time playing it, they become very proficient and travel all over Europe, and even Ireland, exhibiting their prowess and stamina on the field during the daytime and rewarding the local female population with their surfeit of afternoon energy in the evening.

If a student survives his first three years of study, when he is about as close to the actual study of medicine as is a man who runs a car wash to being an automobile engineer, he sits his second M.B. examination and, if successful, is allowed to enter the actual world of medicine and start working in hospital wards and dealing with patients.

Rugby and sex will sometimes make it necessary to take three or four attempts at this examination, which is the requirement for allowing the metamorphosis to take place.

To distinguish the hospital medical student from the rest of the medical staff, he is equipped with a short bum-freezer white coat. As this is also the uniform of the hospital porter and male kitchen staff, it does allow the student to do a bit of portering if he gets bored, and kitchen work if he gets cold and hungry. Similarly, it enables porters and embryo chefs to join in on ward rounds and, in later years, for them to set up medical advice centres and abortion clinics.

Obstetrics

Here you not only have to deliver twenty babies before you get your card signed, but have to wash up as well. I just can't believe that infant mortality is on the decrease, particularly in teaching hospitals. I did find, if I picked out the more elderly fertile woman who had already gone through this particular experience five or six times, that my part in the delivery was little different than taking a short sharp angled pass from a rugby scrum. I only ever dropped one baby and that was when the mother sneezed at the moment of delivery.

Casualty Department

In the Casualty Department a student learns to stitch and put on Plaster-of-Paris casts, often with little supervision, and here they tend to do their own thing. I earned a severe reprimand for doing a buttonhole stitch on a Jamaican navvy, and my first three leg plasters were so heavy that the patients all slipped a disc when they tried to move their encased limbs.

Playing It Cool

When a medical student is let into the hospital for the first time, unless he was a patrol leader or something in the Boy Scouts and took his First Aid Badge, he will have no knowledge of medicine at all. For some (just a few) the first female breast they have to examine will be the nearest they have been to this particular organ since they were weaned. Nevertheless, they have to appear to act with dignified aplomb in spite of their bum freezers and give the impression that it is all matter of fact and that they have been doing it for years.

At my own first particular appearance in this field I was called from the back of the round of thirty or so students to examine the right hand side of the chest of an attractive dark haired woman of about twenty-eight who was having some trouble in that region. Never having approached a female in this situation before, I reached out with my shaking groping fingers to the

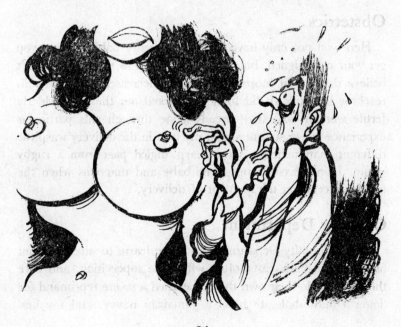

afflicted organ to have them smacked away by the female patient with : 'That's enough of that' as soon as I made contact. I was not helped by rustic comments of 'sexy' and 'beast' by my associates or the chiding of the physician who was conducting the round for being too clumsy. After that I always ducked down on ward rounds and didn't examine anybody again properly until after I had qualified.

Tit for Tat

Three months later, determined to get my own back on the physician who had put me in this humiliating position, I was given a golden opportunity when he called for a chair to elaborate a point at a bedside consultation. Only on getting up after he had finished his dissertation and diagrams did he realise I had fetched him a commode.

As a student one spends a few months in each of many departments of the hospital.

Surgery

Surgery, for me, meant hours of pulling on retractors and, as the patient was covered in sheets with tubes going in at both ends, I never knew which end was which. Being poor at anatomy, for several months my surgical experience led me to believe that the stomach and intestines lay directly above the heart. It was a great shock one day when they lifted the sheets off a patient before he left the theatre and I found I had been pointing the wrong way.

Medicine

Medical wards, long routines of note taking and listening to chests with stethoscopes. We found the stethoscope was the ideal communal drinking instrument. If the bell, the lower end, were lowered into the standard beer pint, two students could sup quite happily through the available ear pieces and talk out of the side of their mouths at the same time. After one such luncheon refreshment, having taken a most careful detailed history of my next

35

patient, who was a stockbroker friend of the consultant physician, I began my examination by laying my stethoscope on his chest, only to see a trickle of beer begin to percolate through the undergrowth that lay between his nipples. My plea of a new type of cleaning fluid was not accepted.

Gynaecology

One of the most testing, emotional times for medical students. It is during this particular course that many become so disillusioned by life in general that they chuck up the whole thing and become monks.

It was during gynaecology that our class idiot reached the peak of his career. Leaning forward, doing a particularly personal type of internal examination in the Gynaecology Outpatient Clinic on some poor, unfortunate female patient, he was so engrossed with his two finger assessment that he was slack about his way of approach and, on standing back on completion of his examination, found that the end of his tie was stuck in the particular orifice that had been under observation.

Ward Rounds

Perhaps the most tedious part of medical student life; wandering around in groups, spending interminable hours listening to droning case histories over patients' bedsides. Something has to be done to relieve this boredom, and there are a number of distractions which are used to while the afternoon away.

1. With one eye on the lecturer conducting the round, with the other eye mentally undress each nurse as she trips about the ward doing her routine work. It is important to keep your mind exactly divided during this exercise because, if the two halves are allowed to mix, you could be called out of your reverie by the lecturer: 'What do you think about this abdominal tumour, Jones?' The answer: 'A black brassiere' only confuses.

2. Sabotage. Go round blocking up stethoscope tubes with bits of plasticine. This means that even the brightest student can't hear anything when he listens in, and of the twenty people in your group you will find that five then go and see a hearing

36

specialist because they think they are going deaf, and the other fifteen will go out and have their ears syringed.

3. Always volunteer to go and fetch instruments, charts, etc., when they are requested, and come back with the wrong thing. When asked, for example, to fetch a receiver (which is a small, kidney-shaped bowl used for putting in swabs, syringes, etc.), bring back a bed pan. When asked to fetch clips (which are used for all sorts of procedures) come back with bicycle clips, and when asked what possible use these objects are in medicine, reply with as straight a face as possible that someone had told you they were very useful in the treatment of diarrhoea.

4. Put sugar lumps in every specimen of urine you can find, then some Professor will write a paper on this strange epidemic of sugar diabetes.

5. Make offensive smells. Many students have the ability to produce these on demand, but the more refined will have to rely on small glass ampules purchased from joke/trick gift shops. This procedure is always useful in breaking up groups.

6. Faint. Not only does this bring the round to an abrupt halt, but gives you credit bonuses because, although you have spent the last two months alternately boozing and attending the Hammersmith Palais, if you faint on a ward round it will be assumed you have been spending the sleeping hours bashing the books. The Dean of the Medical School will call you in and tell you to ease up, making a note of your industry and application.

Outpatients

Outpatients are less boring than Ward Rounds because, if you can find a hypodermic syringe and receiver, all you have to do is to walk round with a purposeful look on your face and it will be assumed that you are just about to do something, and there is every chance you will be able to slip away and play a hand of cards with the outpatients' porters.

Some of the happiest hours for medical students are spent in the V.D. Clinic. There is no doubt the clientele are friendly and sociable, and one learns hitherto unknown facts of life, like why cucumbers should be peeled, etc.

On through all the specialties—ear, nose and throat; skins; plastic surgery; orthopaedics; then one day, after several tries, it is all over. Medical students suddenly become doctors, and wish they had at least learnt something before they had this responsibility thrust upon them. Memories are all that is left of those happy, carefree days.

The Great Life

Medicine plays only a small part in the medical student's life. It is the other freedoms and achievements that most miss. As well as rugby and sex, drinking and dancing have taken up a large part of the student's leisure time. They live either in hostels, digs, or grotty, over-populated unhygienic flats, littered with skeletons, empty beer bottles, road signs and dirty washing up.

Colleagues of mine, now famous physicians and surgeons, achieved greater fame by placing a chamber pot on both the Albert Memorial and the House of Commons during the same night.

One student, who had zoo contacts, could arrange animals for all occasions—elephants for the rugby cup final, a tiger for the hospital dance, and a camel for yet another hospital rugby match. With the knowledge that the Queen would be attending the next Championship Final, something special had to be arranged. Two elephants were ordered, then a last minute cancellation—one had come into season, and no risks could be taken. Missing the climax of the possibility of having two elephants mating on the touch-line before Royalty was too much for this particular student, who gave up medicine and became a trapeze artist.

Many students spend much of their time as film extras, some as dance-room stewards, and one as a chucker-out in a strip club; all occupations to broaden the mind and understanding of the embryo physician. Approximately 95 per cent of time was spent in this type of occupation, and 5 per cent on medicine, thus ensuring a smooth end product.

A few spend their time hitchhiking through Europe, living on currency manipulations, and a small number (very small) spend their time in the hospital library reading up diseases with unpronounceable names. In the end, the 60 per cent who survive line up to get their degrees and diplomas. Most have just qualified with a minimum of effort, husbanding their energies for the years ahead.

The final qualification party with one inebriated student, having passed his midwifery examination at the fifth attempt, inspired by his success, tried to deliver a booking clerk through the hole in the window at Paddington Station.

Thus students become qualified as doctors, realising that qualifications are only a means to an end, the starting point, and not the finishing line, and this is probably how things should be.

CHAPTER FOUR

General Practitioners

IN ENGLAND nowadays it is difficult to get near a General Practitioner. Whereas, before, they used to wear tweed suits, work in one room, and go fishing on Wednesday afternoons, nowadays they work in groups in large concrete block buildings called Health Centres, guarded by hatchet-faced receptionists. They wear dark suits, sometimes white coats, have flashy cars, and play golf on Sundays. The H.F.Rs (hatchet-faced receptionists) prevent all but a few patients getting through to them, so they spend most of their time stuck by themselves in a room with only *The Times* crossword to do, and tend to put on weight.

The patients, meanwhile, are told that Dr. Brown hasn't an appointment free for the next two weeks, and are advised to go and see what the chemist can offer them.

General Practitioners do still visit people at home when they are sick, and also go out on emergency calls.

The situation in America is similar only in some aspects. There all General Practitioners work from what they call 'offices'. They have an S.S.R. (sweet, smiling receptionist) guarding them, because all patients are potential customers and a tonsillectomy could be the price of a ticket to the Bahamas. They will not visit at home and patients, however ill, have somehow to get to the 'office'.

The place not to be ill in is a certain Middle East country, where there are only three medical schools, and a great shortage of doctors. If you have no money there is no problem—you get no medicine or medical treatment. If you do have money it is not always a great help because, if you perforate your stomach or burst your appendix, there is no rushing into hospital with sirens screaming, it's 'Let's be stoical' till the next morning, when friends or relations have to queue for you at the local hospital to see if a bed is likely to become available that day.

In China all the G.P.s are so busy reading Chairman Mao's Little Red Book that they have little surplus time to attend patients at all.

In France what ills there are are usually associated, or thought to arise from, bad plumbing of the bedroom bidet. When ill it is a 50 : 50 chance whether you send for the plumber or the doctor —usually the first one available suffices.

General practice is an art. You could send a boy to art school to be taught how to paint. Whether he becomes an artist or not depends, not on his instruction, but his flair for expressing himself. Much the same can be said of general practice and General Practitioners.

Some of the arts actually originate in general practice. Not the least of these is the art of 'not listening'.

The Art Of Turning a Deaf Ear

There is no doubt that 'not listening' is an art, and the General Practitioner, by the very nature of his work, is in one of the most favourable circumstances to perfect it.

Like so many other things, it can be made to look easy by the expert, and it is only when it is done in a careless or slipshod fashion that the dangers and pitfalls become obvious.

The skilled artist sits in his surgery with an acquired pleasant, smiling, intense, concentrated look on his face. He asks his first question, and gathers from the patient, say a Mrs. Smith, that she has a pain in her abdomen. He enquires about the nature and history of the pain, and Mrs. Smith answers, 'Well it was the day before my aunt came to stay, and it was raining . . .' etc.

At this stage the artist immediately switches about three-quarters of his mind out of the window, leaving only a few auditory fibres in contact with the ensuing babble, ready to switch fully back again if they pick up a relevant word, such as 'bleeding' or 'vomit', or if they register that the flow has temporarily stopped, and another question is required.

In this way you can see forty people in the morning surgery, deal with their wants, and at the same time work out your income tax, plan your next summer holiday, and compose an after-dinner speech for the Rotary Lunch.

It is most distressing to see the artist who is past his prime, or just over confident, since it is only by constant attention to detail that any degree of skill can be maintained.

When the more specialised branches of the medical profession try to intrude on these general practice skills, they are unaware of the many pitfalls.

Recently a Consultant Physician (a man whom I had previously admired) walked up to a woman patient in out-patients, and said:

'How is your husband getting on, Mrs. Green?'

'But, Dr. X, you know he died three weeks ago—you were looking after him,' she replied.

'Good, well done,' said our Consultant, patting her on the shoulder, 'keep it up,' and he walked out of the room.

Choosing Your Doctor

Most people at some time have dealings with General Practitioners. How you decide on which General Practitioner you visit must be given a lot of thought.

Your choice of doctor depends very much on your personal taste. This may be for one old and comforting, who can always be relied upon to give you a bottle of medicine and an off-work note, or one of these new busy young doctors who are always sticking needles into you and shoving instruments up unnatural places, who send you back to work, not because you are feeling better, but because your blood count is normal.

Many decide according to the abundance and colour of the hair, or even the lack of it, whilst for others what car he is driving is the deciding factor.

For a time German doctors became very popular for the piercing way they used to look at you.

Choosing is made much easier nowadays because, far from deciding who will look after you, it's very difficult to find anyone to take you on at all. All one can do is to try and make a friend of the particular one with whom you are lumbered.

General Practitioners are often very interesting people. They always go abroad for their holidays, win prizes for vegetables at local horticultural shows (usually grown by their gardeners who come in once a week), are connoisseurs of food and wine and, whatever their income, usually have an overdraft.

They practise medicine in two different ways.

Keep Taking The Tablets

The first group give you masses of bottles of medicine and tablets whatever the reason for your visit. This is fine if you are not feeling ill, or if you want the coloured tablets for your Ludo set. But if, for example, you came in to have your passport photo signed, you might begrudge the subscription charges you are forced to pay for the medicine that is thrust upon you.

The Psychological Kick

The second group don't give medicines at all. They believe in talking to you. The most you will ever get out of them is a grudging aspirin. Unfortunately, this group decide what is wrong with you as you come through the door, don't let you get a word in edgeways, talk for half an hour, then send you out, being very pleased with themselves, considering that they can notch up another cure.

That the numbers attending surgeries of this group get smaller and smaller doesn't worry them. They put this up as proof that they are curing people, not realising that all the dissatisfied patients are leaving for another practice, or consulting with the junior partner.

One of the most successful general practitioners I know diagnosed cerebral tumours in most of his patients, pointing out to them how lucky they were to have come to him because he had tablets that would shrivel the tumours up. He would then give them the tablets, and arrange to see them again in a month's time. At this next appointment he would examine them, and pronounce them cured.

Nobody was ever able to prove him wrong. He had a 100 per cent cure rate, and there is one small corner of England where half the population is walking about with cured cerebral tumours. It must be something in the water.

Alas, this particular practitioner came to an untimely end because, following some trouble with his eyes and having persistent headaches, he died of a cerebral tumour.

Another practitioner installed a machine in his surgery for giving electric convulsions. Whatever conditions his patients presented him with, be it asthma, rheumatic arthritis or gout, before leaving they had to submit themselves to a convulsion. Strangely, most of them got better.

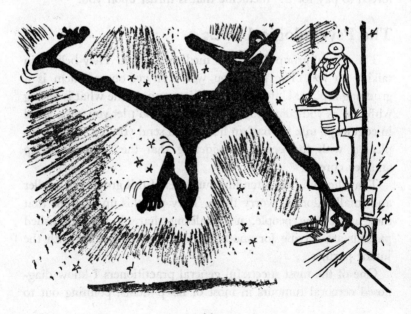

New Drugs For Old Pains

In the good old days all there was to offer was pink or green medicine, which the doctor made up at the sink while you waited, and everybody kept well. Now, with the ever increasing number of drug house representatives pressing samples on the General Practitioner, you never know what might be pressed upon you that the Doctor is trying out. The adage 'It's bound to be good—the advertisements speak well of it' being much to the fore.

A few stick to old-fashioned remedies such as bronchitic children being sent out to breathe the fumes whilst they are tarring the road, but by-and-large pills, pills, pills.

An American who carried a special jewelled pill box with rows of different types of pills was asked what he did when he didn't know which pill to take. 'Oh,' he replied, 'there is a special pill for that contingency.'

There was a scheme suggested that drug house representatives should be made to take their own preparations for two months before they started to market them. There are so many new preparations, however, that the idea was dropped as impracticable.

General Practitioners' surgeries used to be dusty old rooms with stuffed horsehair examination couches. They have now changed to bright, clinical monstrosities, bristling with syringes, needles and other instruments of torture.

Each General Practitioner is allowed, under the National Health Service, to look after up to a maximum of 3,500 patients. This means that, if your practice is in Torquay, you look after 1,000 patients and become very wealthy : if your practice is in spitting distance of Wigan Pier, you will have 10,000 patients on your list and die of a coronary at the age of thirty-five.

General Practitioners are the backbone of the medical profession, acting as a clearing house for the more specialised branches of medicine, keeping and looking after all but a very small percentage of the unwell, and dealing with them each in his own inimitable way.

There is no such thing as a normal General Practitioner. The range of difference is so great that an Evangelical Missionary and a Witch Doctor would both be accepted in the common run.

A College and A Coat Of Arms

Recently there has been an effort to get General Practitioners to look more respectable by having their own College Coat of Arms, and issuing their own diplomas. This has been a great deal of fun for a lot of people.

Any General Practitioner who passes the examination of this august body can use the letters M.C.G.P. after his name, thus preventing General Practitioners having inferiority complexes when they sit down to dinner with M.R.C.P.s and F.R.C.S.s etc.

I have never quite understood what the initials mean, but assume it is something like Motorised Chinese Girl Policewomen. These letters can be attained, as mentioned earlier, by passing an exam or by having paid a subscription at the very beginning. By definition this was so long ago that the recipients have already forgotten all the medicine they ever knew, and it is this body who examines the incoming potential Girl Policewomen.

The more distinguished members of the College write lots of erudite papers on illness surveys, usually on groups of three or four people, showing that they have not quite got rid of their inferiority complex with M.R.C.P.s and F.R.C.S.s.

This is all—apart from being good fun—a great waste of time. General Practitioners do not need to know any medicine— they need no other instrument than the pen. They don't have inferiority complexes when dining with specialists nowadays because they earn very much more money and can appear in cars twice the size, and smoke big Havana cigars after dinner. And if you want a few more letters after your name, all you have to do is to get your uncle to put you up for membership of the Royal Commonwealth Society and, overnight, you are entitled to put the letters F.R.C.S. after your name (Fellow of the Royal Commonwealth Society).

CHAPTER FIVE

House Surgeons

House surgeons, as explained later in the book, can be recognised by their white coats and inability to communicate in English. They, like all other types of doctor, come in every hue, shape and size. Black countries tend to have white House Surgeons; white countries black House Surgeons; yellow countries, red House Surgeons; and red countries, yellow House Surgeons.

There was a time when there was an attempt by yellow House Surgeons to invade America, but as there are so many enthusiastic General Surgeons in America itching to have a go at anything, anybody yellow was immediately investigated to find some medical cause for their skin colour, and yellow House Surgeons fled back to Yellowland, many leaving their gall bladders behind them.

Bricks And Mortar Don't Need Surgeons

House Surgeons in the main are not House Surgeons at all. Real House Surgeons, to be true to the name, drive a bulldozer and knock down rows of old terrace houses. This type of House Surgeon has little part to play in the general run of hospital life although we once nearly called one in to someone who hadn't opened his bowels for three weeks. They can be distinguished from Hospital Doctor House Surgeons by the fact that they drive Ford Cortinas, go to the Costa Brava for their holidays, and have lots of money; whilst Hospital House Surgeons just go to sleep on their holidays and don't have any money at all.

Tree Surgeons fall half-way between these two categories, and can be called in for advice both on houses and hospital patients.

'House Surgeon' is the name given to junior hospital doctors, irrespective of which branch of medicine they are involved in. Only a few will be in any way connected with surgery. It is the first post you have after qualifying, and in most countries now you have to spend a couple of years at one of these posts before being allowed out to practise on your own. It is really the peak of your medical career.

House Surgeons are more knowledgeable than any other type of doctor, will have a go at anything, whatever the risk (unless it's to themselves), and whatever else they do after their time on the House it's always a downhill journey of both performance and confidence. That this should be the peak of their medical attainment is quite understandable, since in England they had done nothing but play Rugby for six years; in America, they have had seven years of hard rioting; in France they have been sleeping with older women for seven years, and are now qualified to try younger ones; and in China they have been hard at it with Mao's Little Red Book.

Armed with this knowledge, they are unleashed on the general public and have to be got past, round, through, before you can receive any other medical opinion or treatment in a hospital.

Training varies from country to country, and Casualty Departments—which are the main ports of entry to hospitals— are full of House Surgeons, and it is in Casualty Departments that the national traditions of treatment are the most clearly demarcated. Suppose, for example, you are involved in a traffic accident resulting in both legs being amputated and a heavy loss of blood.

In France they would pull your trousers down to see if your vital organs had been involved. No treatment would be started until a celebratory glass of cognac had been drunk all round to mark that the accident had in no way impaired your ability to fire on both cylinders.

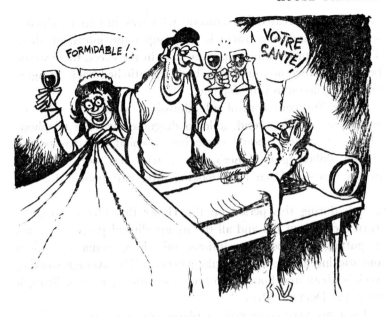

Patients' Qualifications For Treatment

In America, before anyone would touch you, you would first
have to prove beyond doubt that you could financially afford
the treatment that you might have to have.

In England you would be asked which school you went to.
A good Public School with First 15 Colours at Rugby would
mean that the orthopaedic consultant surgeon would be down
to see you within two minutes : a Grammar School and a Degree
at a red-brick university would mean that the Registrar (who is
half-way between a House Surgeon and a Consultant) would be
down in fifteen minutes; and a Secondary Modern School, and
a supporter of Leyton Orient, would probably mean being
shoved into a side room and left until the next duty shift took
over.

In China, of course, they would just read you the first ten
pages of Chairman Mao's Little Red Book.

Happily many hospital porters have first-aid certificates and
can cope with most things; or you might even be fortunate

enough to be treated by someone who was just in to pinch a white coat, and since there is no group more informed about TV medical programmes than the man in the street, there would be every chance of you having both legs stitched back on again and being home in time for tea.

House Surgeons control all admissions to hospital and are always, in a split second, able to diagnose over the telephone whether a patient should come into hospital, this irrespective of the skilled practitioner's views, who has been qualified twenty years and has been looking after this patient for two months.

It is during this period on the House that House Surgeons learn the facts of life and all the minor clinical procedures such as putting up blood transfusions, injections, minor operations and sticking needles into people generally. The average working week is about 200 hours, 180 hours of which are spent living it up in the Doctors' Mess.

These are very cosmopolitan places nowadays and the House staff that I worked with consisted of two Poles, three Indians, one Pakistani, one Lebanese, one Chinese, five Irish and myself. I always used to keep my passport in my left hand front pocket in case of accident.

Registrars

After a few years as a House Surgeon (or Houseman, as they are called, whether male or female) at last comes the day when the young Hospital Doctor has to make a decision as to what to do about the future. All House Surgeon appointments are for six months and in time he will have explored all the jobs available and, knowing him, nobody will touch him the second time round. This exploring can take some years because, like everything else, there are countless types of Housemen—there are surgical ones; paediatric; gynaecological; pathological (many of these); obstetrics; ear, nose and throat; medical; neurological; dermatological; anaesthetic; casualty; thoracic; orthopaedic; and even fine divisions like surgical/paediatric; medical/paediatric, to name but a few.

Long Hours And A Lot To Drink

This life of no money, long hours and too much booze has to stop though, like picking your nose, it's a difficult habit to finish with.

There are two main options open. One is to go into immediate wealth as a General Practitioner, the other is to stay on in hospital as a Hospital Doctor, with prolonged penury, but with the vision, the fame and success in the very far distance.

As this chapter is about Hospital Doctors, the House Surgeons who chicken out and go into General Practice will have to go off and find a chapter of their own.

Hospital Doctors who have passed the caterpillar stage of being a House Surgeon now chrysalise for a few years (six to forty) into what is known as Registrars before they burst out in the full glory of butterflies (Consultants).

A Registrar is a more serious Hospital Doctor than a House Surgeon, and does all the practical work in the hospital, kept going by the fact that, one day, he might become a Consultant (Specialist), when he will have all his own work done by other Registrars. The term 'Registrar' is a dubious one. Don't, for example, go to a Registrar of Births and Deaths and ask him to remove your appendix. He will almost certainly try, with a good chance of you requiring one of his other two departments. Registrars all wear baggy trousers, down-at-heel shoes, and larger stethoscopes than House Surgeons. They turn up the collars of their white coats; that is, of course, until they become Senior Registrars (there are of course Junior, Middle and Seniors), when they start to practise wearing pin-stripe trousers, stiff white collars, Club ties, and clean their cars on Sunday mornings. There is no doubt they do all the work, and this is where they acquire all their medical knowledge.

Operation Successful?

Most hospital operations are carried out by Registrars, and if it is your misfortune to go into hospital for an operation, it is almost certainly a Registrar who will do it. So, if you wake up and find he has grafted a kidney under your left arm, or coupled your waterworks to your knees, be patient with him—this is probably his first solo with a knife. And also this is how many original medical discoveries are made. You might become a special case and be used in demonstrations, and think how useful it would be if you could pass water through your knees, particularly at football matches.

Registrars are always serious, busy, walk about reading learned papers, and writing papers about their own discoveries. Much of their time is spent on research. It was a Registrar who did all the groundwork on the surgery of grasshoppers. Grasshoppers were taught to jump on the word of command—they could do it like Guardsmen. This Registrar then cut the back legs off all the grasshoppers, and he noticed that, after the operation, they no longer obeyed the command to jump even when thrashed with matchsticks, thus making the startling discovery that if you cut off a grasshopper's back legs, it can no longer hear. Then there was the chance discovery by a Medical Registrar (yes, they have all the sub-divisions) demonstrating the effects of alcohol to a group of medical students. He placed a worm in a beaker of water, showing the students being lectured how it swam around happily and freely but, when placed in a beaker of gin, the worm died instantly, thus proving if you drink enough gin you will never have worms.

Afraid Of Nothing

Registrars are afraid of nothing and will tackle any surgery from a circumcision to plastic surgery. One more intelligent than most used the waste product of the first of these two operations as material for eyelids in his plastic work. Although his colleagues prophesied that he would finish up with a lot of cock-eyed patients, in fact he found that he had endowed most of them with foresight.

Registrars learn how to cut off legs, how to stitch them back on again if they cut off the wrong leg by mistake, how to graft, both surgically and financially, and are always rushing round doing special blood and urine tests on people. The fact that they look so serious is not because they are worried about their patients, but they are worrying about their house mortgage, their increasing number of children and, ultimately, whether they will ever be able to leave it all behind and become a Consultant. They can't wait to dry their wings in the sun.

Some make it, others become disgruntled General Practitioners. Most go abroad and finish off as Professor of Surgery in all sorts of unheard of parts of the world.

CHAPTER SIX

Surgeons

IT IS THE initial dream of every doctor to become a Surgeon. The drama, the money, and the absolute power of being able to chop bits out of people as you feel. It is no easy path to reach this exalted position, and one has already had years sitting about as a House Surgeon or Registrar (as described in the previous chapter) before one can finally become a Consultant Surgeon. Many fall by the wayside, and the ones that do eventually make it are always marked by this exacting apprenticeship and have the time to develop peculiar eccentricities.

Surgeons Galore

In this day and age 'Consultant Surgeon' is too wide a term to use, because with so much specialisation there are no general surgeons left. When sending for one, you have to ask for the specific type you want. To name but a few—there are Eye Surgeons, Ear Surgeons, Nose Surgeons, Bladder Surgeons, Stomach Surgeons, Leg Surgeons, Arm Surgeons, Back Surgeons, Hand and Foot Surgeons, Brain Surgeons, and Plastic Surgeons. The term 'Plastic Surgeon' does not mean a Surgeon who is made of plastic, which is the obvious translation, nor does it mean a Surgeon who plays with plasticine; it means a Surgeon who carries out plastic operations on other people.

Then there are a few who specialise in small parts of one field, like a man who does nothing but remove bunions, and one who

I know who does nothing else but operate on haemorrhoids (piles). The latter is always a danger at a party, because at the mere hint of someone toasting 'Bottoms up', he is straight away reaching for his scalpel.

The most successful of all Surgeons is one who specialises in things like varicose veins, chopping the veins out, a bit at a time, knowing that nature will replace the removed piece in a fairly short space of time. Thus, if he can enrol a list of about twenty-four wealthy patients, he knows that he has a steady living for life.

There is of course great social grading, depending on the type of Surgeon you are, with Brain Surgeons at the very top of the scale, and of course Pile, or Haemorrectomy Surgeons, at the bottom.

The Name Of The Game

It is very important for Surgeons to have operations named after them, and they spend a lot of time thinking about different ways to do things. If, for example, a Surgeon called Jones found that the easiest way to remove a spleen was from the left-hand side of the body, the region where the spleen actually lies, the operation would then be called 'Jones' Operation' or, for the highly educated, 'A Jones' splenectomy', since adding 'ectomy' to any word just means taking it out, hence appendicectomy means taking out the appendix, nephrectomy means removing the kidney, and fingerectomy means pulling your finger out. Everybody will write learned papers about it, and Jones will write a book saying how he first thought about it, and dedicate the book to his wife.

A Surgeon called Brown will then do the operation from the right-hand side, which is much further away, and is much more difficult to perform. It has no advantages, and many disadvantages over Jones' operation, but Brown is damned if he is going to be up-staged by an idiot like Jones, who didn't even go to a good medical school. Hence Brown's operation will be born with subsequent papers and the proverbial book.

This will be followed by Smith's operation, where you will

approach it from above; Jenkins' operation, where you approach it from below; and Carruthers' operation, where you approach it from the back.

Apart from the papers and the books, to advertise their particular approach each Surgeon will invent some new surgical instrument to facilitate his particular operation, this series of operations resulting in Smith's square retractors, Jones' round retractors, Brown's long-toothed forceps, Jenkins' short-toothed forceps, and Carruthers' non-toothed forceps.

More and More Instruments

Every Theatre Sister in the land will have to learn five new surgical instruments, and if she wants to go to an early, untimely end, all she has to do is, in the heat of a major operation, give Surgeon Smith a Jones' retractor, or Surgeon Jenkins Carruthers' non-toothed forceps.

Eventually a man called Dr. Polanski, who has given this operation a lot of thought, will say that the condition should be treated conservatively, i.e. do nothing about it and hope it will go away. This term has nothing to do with the Conservative Government, but on second thoughts, it easily could. Polanski will be knighted and a special paragraph will be included about him in all medical textbooks.

At this stage the Physicians will poke their noses into the chapter on Surgeons and say better results are achieved if the patient treated by the Polanski method is put on a bran diet. The condition will then become a medical one and be treated with bran and bed rest until whatever it is that is being treated bursts. Then a Surgeon called White will be called in, who will operate from the left side, the side nearest the organ, and remove the burst spleen. He will write papers about it, a book about it, and this operation will also produce a White's pressure sponge holder.

Then a Surgeon called Black will operate for a burst spleen from the right side, the side furthest away from the organ, the papers and books will be produced, Black's rounded artery forceps will be invented, and so on, and so on, and so on.

A Little Bit Here, A Little Bit There...

At a medical school reunion one middle-aged doctor approached one of his immaculately dressed contemporaries, saying 'Hello, Ponsonby-Jones, what are you doing with yourself nowadays?' 'Actually,' said Ponsonby-Jones, 'I am a Brain Surgeon.' 'I always knew you would do well,' said the first doctor, 'you were always the brightest in our year, but isn't it frightfully difficult?' 'No,' said Ponsonby-Jones, 'quite simple actually. A ligature here, a snip there, and Bob's your uncle. But, tell me, dear fellow, what are you doing yourself?' 'Nothing very much,' said the first doctor, 'I specialise in sex change surgery.' 'Surely,' said Ponsonby-Jones, 'that must have its difficulties?' 'Not a bit,' said the first doctor, 'a ligature here, a snip there, and Bob's your aunt.'

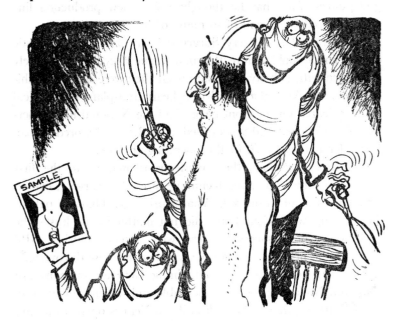

A Spare Part Man

Transplant surgery has recently added a new vista to this particular field. Nothing is impossible any more—there are spare parts for anything, and if you don't happen to be carrying one yourself, you can always borrow one from your sister or uncle. You can have new hearts, lungs, livers, kidneys. You name it, the Surgeons have got it. It's even worse than plastic surgery, where they could change the shape of things; now wear something out, and it can always be replaced. When you go to the Bank nowadays the odds are that you don't go to cash a cheque but to see if they have any colons your size in stock.

Transplant surgery, like all other forms of life, is prone to blackmailing and the falling of standards. This particular form of surgery was briefly popular for men who felt that Nature had not endowed them with enough masculine equipment. All was well until one day a middle-aged gentleman, sporting his new 500-guinea model, noticed his old one being worn by his grocer in a gentlemen's convenience, the grocer having paid 300 guineas for what he thought was a new production line model. Greed is the end of so many of us.

Since transplant surgery Surgeons have undergone a drastic change in outlook. Before this new vogue they were relatively quiet men with nobody quite sure what they were doing. All this has changed. After the first British heart transplant the surgical team appeared on the front page of all the National newspapers with fists clenched and arms raised, as if they had scored a goal. I wonder if they kissed in the operating theatre?

Not to be outdone, the Americans treated us to the first attempt at a new operating technique of cardiac surgery, live on TV. We were all enthralled. What a privilege. That the patient died within twenty-four hours did not matter in the least—the operation was a success. There were queues outside GPs' surgeries the next day for people wanting this new discovery.

Alas, the last of the few remaining General Surgeons are dying off. No longer are there men able and willing to have a go at anything anywhere. Nowadays if a patient is opened up, and the opening Surgeon finds the bit that needs to be operated on is lower down than the bit he specialises in, the operation is halted until the Surgeon who specialises in the lower-down bit is found. This specialisation has even spread to people who take things like x-rays. Once, stuck in the middle of the Sahara with

58

a stone in my kidney, the only other doctor in the party (an American lady) couldn't give me a pain-relieving injection because all her job entailed was illustrating the contents of the abdomen with dyes in the bloodstream. She was an abdominal angiographist. We can't even afford them over here.

But in spite of all this gloom, it's all marvellous. If you can afford it, you can have your toes transplanted on to your hands, and your fingers transplanted to your feet, the only disadvantage being that it is now possible to contract athlete's foot shaking hands, and the sight of somebody picking their nose with their feet is absolutely appalling.

The following list outlines the duties of the Specialists who come under the heading of 'Surgeons'. It is hoped that this will be of some help to the reader.

(a) **Orthopaedic Surgeons.** They, as yet, have not been too swayed by transplant surgery, but have learnt these new techniques of nailing limbs back on. At whatever age now, if you break your leg, you have it hammered back with a nail before you can say 'Jack Robinson'. The only disadvantage is that, if you are on a plane or ship, you may affect the magnetic compass and land hundreds of miles from your destination.

(b) **Thoracic Surgeons.** They confine their surgery to opening chests, so if you have an old chest padlocked away in your cupboard for many years and can't open it, a Thoracic Surgeon is your man.

(c) **Eye Surgeons.** Eye Surgeons, as supposed, operate on eyes. They get so confined with this small field they have been heard to exclaim, 'It's all a lot of b—ls'.

(d) **E.N.T. Surgeons** are not men who just operate on males and tea bags. E.N.T. stands for 'Ear, Nose and Throat', and if you find this book hard to swallow, these are the people to approach.

(e) **Genito-urinary Surgeons** deal with any surgery applied to the waterworks. They are in some way affected by their work; a few have webbed feet, all are good swimmers, and most own a yacht.

59

(f) **Gynaecological Surgeons**—see chapter on Gynaecologists.

(g) **Plastic Surgeons.** Plastic Surgeons, as mentioned earlier, do not work with plasticine, but will shape or reshape any part of the body you desire. One patient, having a nose remade, half-way through the process discharged himself with a roll of flesh running from his forehead to where his nose used to be, and made a good living in a fair from then on as the Elephant Man.

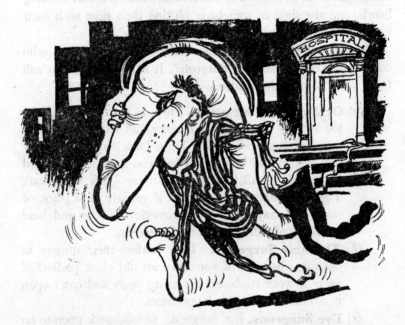

(h) **Renal Surgeons** take out and put back kidneys. They often have a few lying around, so always examine very carefully what you are eating if they ask you out to dinner.

(i) **Cardiac Surgeons** are the glamour boys of the profession and are said to have taken the heart right out of surgery.

(j) **Rectal Surgeons** do unmentionable things to you from behind. One once describing his area of surgery estimated the distance from two points in the alimentary

canal and said, 'As the crow flies . . .' just showing that there is much more going on back there than you ever thought.

A Red And White Pole

Originally all Surgeons were barbers as well and, similarly, all barbers were Surgeons as well. With all the new innovations of transplant, cosmetic, plastic and other types of surgery, we are heading back to the day when Surgeons will have a red and white pole outside their consulting rooms, and it might be possible to order an appendicectomy and a shampoo for the same day

CHAPTER SEVEN

Physicians

It is often difficult for the lay person to understand exactly what a Physician is. I think Physicians often have the same trouble.

Everybody understands what a Surgeon is. They cut people about, and there is a fair understanding that Surgeons sometimes stick to one part of the body and become an Arm or Leg, or Abdominal Surgeon, etc., but Physicians—what on earth do they do?

A Lazy Lot

It would be fair to say that Physicians cope with that part of medicine that isn't covered by surgery or childbirth. This is a very wide field and is, of course, divided into multiple specialities none of which carries out any real practical procedures for their patients. Whereas a Surgeon can be blamed for not taking off a leg properly, or taking the wrong one off, Physicians really don't do anything at all so can never be blamed for anything, and some of the other groups, like Neurologists who come under the same headings, do even less still if that is possible in the carrying out of practical procedures.

When tests are required to be done, like sticking needles into chests and bones, putting up blood transfusions, etc., the Registrars and Housemen have to do these so it is possible for a Physician not to have touched a patient for years.

The Cure To End All Cures

The greatest blow to Physicians was the discovery of antibiotics when, overnight, a number of conditions which had previously been fatal became instantly curable. No more days and nights of hovering over a pneumonia, awaiting the crisis. A handful of pills given by a General Practititoner will reduce it to the status of a cold in the nose.

No Fun No More

Thus all the excitement was taken out of medicine in an instant. Now there were pills which got people better almost straight away. Before these days of antibiotics medicine was great fun. People either got better or they didn't. If they did get better, whatever they were taking at the time was given the credit for having cured them. This is how old wives' cures like tying your left sock round your neck for tonsillitis and rubbing on a snail to reduce your mumps swellings arose. It is possible that Physicians were responsible for most of these.

Before the advent of Penicillin there were two main schools for the treatment of pneumonia. One was the hot treatment—keeping the patient hot, applying poultices (kaolin and linseed) to the chest; the other was the cold treatment—keeping the patient cold and applying ice bags to the chest. What decided whether the patient lived or died of course had nothing to do with the treatment, but much more on things like whether he kept up his daily intake of Guinness when he felt unwell, and whether he was taking his full course of pickled onions.

But pneumonia was a disease to be treated by Physicians, who often at the start of a treatment would immediately stop the two just mentioned staffs of life, endangering the patient from the onset; then, depending on which school they belonged to, would start the hot or cold treatment.

Pneumonia is similar to politics, being usually left or right, depending on whether it is the left or right lung that is affected.

Hot Or Cold

One day a poor unfortunate was admitted to a London teaching hospital with a left lobar pneumonia and was immediately treated with ice bags (the cold treatment) for this particular condition. He survived to the week-end when, as is the wont of teaching hospitals, the Physician in charge of his case went off for two days' golf and all the medical cases came under the care of one of his colleagues, who happened to be one of the foremost advocates for the hot treatment of pneumonia. He could not change the treatment already prescribed by his colleague, but when the patient also developed a right lobar pneumonia in addition to his left (double pneumonia) he dived in straight away on the new side with hot packs and poultices. The patient, despairing of ice packs and poultices being applied to opposite sides of his chest for two hours, and fancying his chance with a nice night nurse, decided to live, managed to get some Guinness and pickled onions smuggled in, and discharged himself after forty-eight hours.

After antibiotics many Physicians went on the dole or signed on as Ship's Doctors, the remaining ones busied themselves with new games and idiosyncracies and became electrically minded, wiring up every patient who came to see them, examining the subsequent tracings, tut-tutting the time away, that before would have been used on ice bags and poultices. They became grave and serious.

One Professor of Medicine developed an ear-lobe tugging approach that will outlast him by many decades. He would make no decision until he had pulled the lobe of his left ear ten to twelve times. Countless budding professors have since emulated him, and if you ever go to a party and notice a man with a left ear lobe bigger than his right, you can bet your bottom dollar he is a Physician.

Out Of The Horse's Mouth

One other Physician started treating whatever condition was referred to him with bran. If the patient got better it was because of the bran; if he didn't, it was because he hadn't been taking it regularly enough. One highly intelligent racehorse owner, realising the position, sent all his stable lads for a consultation, enabling him to feed his complete string for half the winter on National Health Service bran.

Physicians have large cars, rooms in Harley Street, large incomes and lots of children, most of whom, in time, become Physicians themselves. The recent changes in the pattern of Society offer new hope for them. At present the commonest single cause for admission to a hospital medical bed is for the treatment of tablet (drug) overdosage. This arises from two sources:

1. The amount of tablets of every sort kicking around nowadays.
2. There isn't much else to do nowadays.

The treatment of this condition comes under the care of a Physician and the main procedures are to wash out the tablets, which is done by the Houseman or Registrar, then revive the patient. There are two main schools of thought about the reviving of patients. One is the cold water treatment, the other is the hot water treatment: also, a select few have been given bran. Already the dole queues are shorter and there is a shortage of Ships Doctors.

The following list outlines the duties of the Specialists who come under the heading of 'Physicians' (i.e. non-operating specialists). It is hoped that this will be of some help to the reader.

1. **Psychiatrist.** A Psychiatrist has been defined as a sex maniac who has failed the practical. He will listen to all your troubles and blast you with electricity if you begin to bore him. He will tell you all his own troubles if given half a chance.

2. **Venereologists.** Venereologists deal with the social contagious diseases like syphilis, gonorrhoea, etc., a speciality very much on the up. It is believed it was a venereologist who wrote the song 'I was seated one day at the organ', and it was from a Venereologist that

Churchill borrowed the phrase 'Give us the tools and we will finish the job'.

3. **Dermatologist** (skin specialist). The speciality for the man with outside interests because his work never gets him out of bed, his patients rarely get better and he only has to use two preparations—phenobarbitone and steroid ointment.

4. **Neurologist.** Neurologists tend to get on your nerves. All the most intelligent Doctors become Neurologists. Their main function is to tell you that you can't do anything about what you thought you couldn't do anything about.

5. **Ophthalmologist** (eye specialist)—enables you to get your new reading glasses more expensively than any other way.

6. **Chest Specialist**—(a) the man who specialises in diseases of the chest; (b) the man who judges the opposite sex more by the shape of the soft tissue swellings on the front of the female rib cage than the shape of the female undercarriage (group name 'Bristolians').

And the final group—

7. **Pathologists**—men who work by dead reckoning.

No Cuts For Profit

The way medicine is practised varies from country to country, this being particularly so of Physicians. America which, as always, has the best and worst of everything, has the lead in style and expense. Before a patient actually reaches a Physician there, he has to pass an additional test as well as that of showing his ability to pay the fees, viz., that there is nothing a Surgeon could reasonably cut off him for profit.

American Physicians are the wealthiest profession in the land, if not the world, even heading the delightful lovelies who keep open house for male visitors in the back streets of Soho.

Machines Take Over

American Physicians do more investigations on patients than anyone. Every blood, urine test and x-ray possible is carried out on each patient, and the patients, by tradition, have come to expect it. How the patient feels is no longer taken into account. If your tests are all right, you are all right, and a sudden rise in the death rate probably means one of the investigating machines is out of order, and everybody is not so right after all.

Machines in America have got so advanced with artificial kidneys, heart, lung apparatus, superior respiration, that patients are now kept alive long after they are dead : in fact nobody dies any more. It is just decided, at some stage, to switch you off.

British Physicians slowly imitate their American counterparts. British medicine at its very best doesn't quite reach the great heights of the American best, but the general all-round standard is much higher, and we have nothing approaching the American worst. There is not quite the same dependence on investigations as in America and the patient is still consulted about how he feels : whether he feels better or not, but there is no doubt about the trend.

For Better Or For Worse

A recent article about a piece of apparatus called a peak flow-meter clearly points this out. A peak flowmeter simply measures the efficiency of your breathing. You have to blow down it for it to record its result. It was pointed out by the manufacturers that a patient with breathing difficulties could find that a particular preparation made him feel better when, in actual fact, the peak flowmeter showed he was worse, and similarly, a preparation that made him feel worse could be shown by the meter to be actually making him better.

The one small difficulty that could arise is that there just could be occasions when a Physician had not got his peak flowmeter with him, and neither he nor the patient would know whether he was getting better or not. All they would be able to do would be to stick to the manufacturers' adage that he would be worse when he felt better, or better when he felt worse.

I remember from my student days a patient being admitted with severe pain in the lower chest. The Physician found an abnormal wave on his electrocardiogram tracing (suggesting heart trouble) and was still waving his paper diagnosis around long after the House Surgeon had sewn up the obvious perforation hole in the patient's stomach.

Pins And Needles

In China, Physicians are much more practical than their Western colleagues. Acupuncture rules the day, and there is a set of pins to be stuck somewhere for every conceivable disease. If the patient protests and refuses to be cured, there is nothing like a nail in the tongue to quieten him.

France For The Good Life

In France it is all fresh air, courtesy, charm, and glasses of wine. Physicians there tend to wander about in groups discussing their cases over three-hour luncheons, appearing for a brief hour after their siesta before donning white gloves and going to the Opera House.

French Doctors (unlike British Doctors) do not get struck off the Medical Register for going to bed with their patients. If a French lady says, for example, 'At present I am under Professor X for my treatment', she probably is.

By and large the French do not make a fetish of being ill like the British and Americans, and although they have the worst plumbing and lavatories of the four countries mentioned, they are probably the healthiest.

Alas, round the corner for Physicians looms a spectre worse than antibiotics—Computers. Already they have begun to infiltrate into this field. Before long, all that will be needed will be for the patient to feed in his symptoms to this terrible machine, and he will receive the diagnosis and treatment on a ticker-tape. It will be like going to the launderette.

The queues for the dole will lengthen again, as they will for Ships Doctors.

CHAPTER EIGHT

Gynaecologists

GYNAECOLOGISTS, one of the branches of surgery, have a chapter of their own, principally because they keep to such a narrow field of work. They cannot think in any terms beyond the range of their own speciality, and it was a gynaecologist who said to a dentist, 'However do you manage to stick it, spending most of your lifetime looking down people's throats?'

Gynaecologists specialise in the diseases and surgery relative to the reproductive organs of women. To make sure they miss out on nothing, they also look after the child-bearing side called obstetrics and, in fact, all gynaecologists are actually obstetrician gynaecologists.

For some strange reason, or perhaps a very valid reason, there is a higher average of bachelor specialists in gynaecology than any other single surgical speciality.

Love Story

Most women fall in love with their gynaecologist, and it is probably the profusion to choose from that leads to this state of affairs.

That women should fall in love in this way is one of the strangest medical phenomena of all. It compares with the Dover sole falling in love with a fishmonger, as the most common major gynaecological operation is to be filleted, i.e. to have all the working parts removed. The romantic aura that this procedure evolves is incomprehensible. Perhaps they develop the same attitude of mind as the war-time Japanese suicide pilots who took off in 'planes with no undercarriages, knowing they could never land again.

Perhaps the operated-on female patient realises that from post-operation on, wherever she lands her undercarriage cannot complicate her life any more.

Gynaecologists have longer hair at the back than most Specialists, drive open sports cars, play the piano, and are quite the best dressed of all practising doctors. They are fortunate in the fact that, as Gynaecologists, they only have to do one of four types of operation:

1. **Repair.**

   Where they stitch back undercarriages that have become non-retractable.

2. **Hysterectomies.**

   Where they remove the womb. Their approach to this operation is a bit like an angler because, often, the reason for removing the womb is because the patient has what is known as a fibroid. Fibroids are harmless, benign, sometimes rapidly growing tumours of the womb. They can reach incredible sizes, and it has been reported, in some cases where the condition was neglected, that rather than remove the fibroid from the patient, the patient was removed from the fibroid.

   It is of great personal pride to the operator to have some big ones to his credit, and it has been rumoured that there are clubs like 'The 30 lb. Club', similar to that organisation set up by the Sharkfisher men of Looe in Cornwall.

   If there were an equivalent of the 'Anglers' Mail' in the world of gynaecology no doubt there would be a prize and a picture of the womb of the month, the successful surgeon sporting his catch on a pair of forceps.

   It is the commonest topic of conversation and only differs from fishing in that you can't describe the one that got away.

3. **Operations on the tubes.**

This does not mean surgery on the London Underground but a variety of procedures that can be carried out on the tubes that link the ovaries to the womb.

(a) They can be tied off, thus keeping the world population numbers down (sterilisation);
(b) Repaired if they burst. This is usually caused by a developing foetus losing its way and turning left instead of right, and
(c) Removed as an encore to a hysterectomy.

4. **Termination of Pregnancy (abortion).**

Alas, this particular operation, since the relaxing of its procedure, has led to a falling off of standards and ethics of a small number of gynaecologists. Whereas for most surgical procedures you are referred by your General Practitioner to a Specialist Surgeon, often in this particular procedure the whole process starts by approaching a taxi driver at London Airport. The monetary rewards for those who dedicate their lives to this particular operation are tremendous, and next to football pool winners they become the wealthiest in the land.

Lady patients have great faith and confidence in their gynaecologist, ask their advice on nearly all non-medical matters and would willingly submit to having their legs or head cut off if so ordered by their idol.

In the obstetric role the relationship is slightly different. There is still the same love and adulation, but the obstetrician part of the gynaecologist is looked on more as a father figure. Perhaps pregnant mothers do feel paternal. During the nine months of pregnancy, for four weeks the doctor-god lays his (warm, cold, wet, hairy) hand on the expanding abdomen, makes a few clucks, then rushes off to continue his piano practice.

Born In A Field

At nine months the expectant mother, if she can avoid the host of embryo obstetrician gynaecologists (i.e. House Surgeons and Registrars) who are all rushing about trying to get in their quota of Caesarian sections and instrument (forceps) deliveries, will have the baby naturally with only a midwife for company, in much the same way as her counterpart in India will produce her baby at the side of a field, during the lunch hour, in the middle of the corn harvest, returning, undeterred, to do the afternoon shift.

Once delivered of her healthy offspring, the young mother's first positive move is to announce in her local paper her grateful thanks to her obstetrician.

This is the mystique that surrounds obstetrician gynaecologists. Strangely, few of these Specialists take up pot-holing as a hobby. You would think they would do it to keep their hand in. They are devoted to their particular branch of surgery and don't consider any event that is not related to their field of interest is of any importance.

In these days of unisex and sex change surgery, men are already beginning to find their way to the gynaecologist's couch. As yet there is no record of them using the obstetric facilities of the partnership.

It is believed by some that, with their vast experience of working in confined spaces, it will be finally gynaecologists who will be called in to set the Channel Tunnel scheme into operation.

CHAPTER NINE

Patients

PATIENTS are the seeds from which all medicine springs. They are all different, yet in a way similar, as a cross-section of the average waiting room contents, be it Leeds, Long Island or Shanghai, would be very much the same. A balance of the genuine sick, off-beat patients, and the also-runs.

In fact waiting rooms vary more, and can in no way be judged by the quality of the magazines present. Once, on the Tassili Plateau in Algeria, conducting an open-air surgery, I refused to continue until the waiting people had stopped throwing camel dung at each other, and I claim this as some sort of record.

Waiting rooms on the left-hand side of Singapore never close and rate five stars in popularity because they are one of the few places you can smoke your opium pipe in peace. In Shanghai, where acupuncture is the main mode of treatment, nails are left purposely sticking up through some of the benches surrounding the walls of the waiting room, resulting in instant cures for half the patients, cutting down considerably on surgery time.

Surgeries, and hence waiting rooms, have been held in every conceivable place. On the top of the list are public houses, particularly if you are on the drug scene, or if you know it is the only likely place for you to bump into your doctor regularly.

One of the great difficulties for the doctor is coping with the off-beat patients who you are not wishing to discourage from seeking medical attention.

Strange Symptoms

To start the morning surgery after having been up all night conducting an heroic midwifery case, you have to make a tremendous mental adjustment to talk on even terms with the first lady patient who complains of passing sea-anemones in her urine, and the second (usually a constipation martyr) who complains of ants in her wainscoting.

In both these cases I am able to offer some treatment. For the first, to cut out drinking sea-water, and the second is quite happy with a bunch of sennapods and a tin of D.D.T.

My third patient has me completely stumped. He complains that people come and knock him unconscious when he is not looking. He may be right. Other than suggest the family club together and buy him a crash helmet, I have little to offer.

My fourth patient, making his third visit to the surgery this week, now complains that he thinks he has a loose wireless valve in his head. After a long consultation he is satisfied with a note to the wireless hospital run by the local electrician.

A Schedule For Blockage

Colonel Banks next, who now campaigns against his bowels as he did against the Afghan tribesmen in the twenties, is an absolute pushover. We are able to work out a detailed schedule for the next two weeks, to meet with any intestinal hold-up, with both district nurses (expert enema givers) standing by like a reserve battalion.

The Sleepless Spinster

Next an eighty-year-old spinster who hadn't slept all week since I diagnosed the pain in her leg as 'intermittent fornication'. She had brought a note from the Priest as a testimony of her chastity, and was only satisfied when I showed her 'intermittent claudication' written clearly in the medical dictionary.

More difficult still for the doctor is the treating of his own family.

The doctor is a hero in many households, and it has been put on record that some patients say that it is sufficient for me to walk into the sick room to put them halfway on the road to complete recovery.

A Prophet Without Honour

One place that my magic does not seem to hold good, however, is in my own home, where the opinion of the domestic help, the gardener or the woman next door, is much more important than that of the qualified expert.

My own wife consults all the do-it-yourself home health guides, and will tell me exactly what I ought to do for the children. When my mother is staying she expects full details of how I should treat various conditions, then tells me how she thinks her own doctor would have treated them differently. She once even offered to show me how to fill in an International Certificate for smallpox vaccination because she was sure I was doing it quite the wrong way.

Doctors either over-treat or under-treat their own families. There seems to be nothing in between. You will find one doctor's family being attended by a stream of consultant colleagues and having all the rarest complications of simple diseases. Their wives have the most complicated obstetric histories and specialists come to deal with any malady that should befall any of them. The more trivial it is, the deeper the possible significance.

The doctor who under-treats his family will blissfully play cricket with his fourteen-year-old son, not realising that the poor lad whose bowling is off to-day is actually showing the classical signs of lobar pneumonia.

In the casualty department of one hospital I met a middle-aged doctor almost in tears. He had just brought his daughter in, having been unsuccessful in stopping her diarrhoea over a period of four days. She had asked, 'Could I go and see a proper doctor, Daddy?'

Some doctors' children are practically weaned on the different types of antibiotics, and if there were such a thing as a penicillin sandwich it would certainly be part of their regular diet. Others, however, reach the age of twenty-one thinking that aspirin is the only available treatment for any disease.

The real trouble is that to his own family a doctor is just an ordinary person, whereas *real* doctors, they believe, are superior, detached human beings who know all the answers. 'You can tell they are good by the way they look at you, and they, not like daddy, can tell what's wrong from the other side of the room, whereas daddy pushes nasty old spoons and things down your throat and hurts you.'

I once tried to syringe my wife's ears—never again. It was nearly the end of our marriage. She now goes off to the local hospital casualty department. I can't say I was delighted when she developed an ear infection after one of her treatments, but I was very matter of fact when I cleared up the residue of the resulting damage.

Ask The Postman

Over the years my family's lack of confidence has slowly undermined my own. Not only do they think I can't treat them and know nothing, but I am beginning to feel it myself. So, whenever one of my children is ill, we usually describe the symptoms briefly to the postman, who has some experience of first-aid, and he outlines the general principles of treatment needed.

My greatest hurt was when one night, preparing a lecture into a tape recorder on the treatment of child complaints, my wife who had heard every word that I was saying in the next room, came out and said, 'Isn't it terrible—every woman reading or hearing that talk will think how lucky the wife of that doctor must be to have such an understanding man about the house, to know exactly what to do when the children are ill or when they have behaviour troubles. And it's not like that at all.'

I did manage for a time to strike a working arrangement with a colleague in which we looked after each other's families, but the two lots of children got together at school, and soon explained to each other the terrible dangers they were being exposed to.

The only time I ever appear popular in my line of treatment at home is when I decide someone is unfit to go to school— then I am the best doctor in the world. In spite of this my younger son gave me the 'Seaman's Manual of Good Health' for Christmas. It is a book designed to keep you in perfect health if the nearest doctor is a thousand miles away.

In the children's view I am of some use elaborating on *Dr. Finlay's Casebook* or *Emergency Ward 10*, but must never ever criticise *Dr. Kildare*.

My major triumph was when I spotted our dog hadn't got colic, but had started to go into labour after an unnoticed pregnancy. 'Gosh, Dad,' the family chorused, 'you really ought to have been a vet!'

Who Needs Enemies?

That copes with doctors' families, but the next difficulty is doctors' friends.

Most doctors claim that they do not make friends of patients. This I never believe. Doctors do have friends who are patients and there is no doubt that friends who are not patients, if they are really close friends, in time become patients.

Treating one's friends is fraught with difficulty. They have access to the ex-directory telephone number and medical communication with them follows a strange ritual.

It starts with a 'phone call, never asking for a visit, but for advice, and protesting against your going. You, of course, protest just as strongly that you must come, as they are friends, and would never impose, and you go however trivial the complaint, cursing under your breath and swearing that never again will you give your number to anyone.

From the moment you arrive the conversation consists of protests from the friends of how much trouble they are causing you, with equal protests from you saying how little it troubles you, and how glad you are they called you.

The friends, being friends, have listened to you when you have exasperatedly been called out for trivial calls, and are very anxious not to be put into your 'bloody nuisance class'. To reassure them you examine so thoroughly, and look so grave, that they are convinced that not only did they do right in getting in touch, but they would have been criminally negligent if they had decided not to. This ensures that next time they get in touch for much less, as they remember this last time when they hadn't thought it was much and you took it so seriously.

The next part of the ritual is to offer you a huge brandy or whisky, which you do not want (I drink very little at the best of times) but have to drink, because if you didn't they would think you were stuffy and offended for having been called out. Your gardening, or post-luncheon snooze, has been interrupted, and all you want to do is to get back, so you toss the drink down quickly, refuse another, and go off.

Who Does The Favour?

Having accepted the drink the balance of power changes. They no longer feel grateful to you, but rather as if they have done you a favour by giving you such a stiff peg (the drink offered on these occasions is never less than half a tumbler full of neat spirit).

As you leave, you can feel them thinking—'the old doc can put it away nowadays', and in spite of the fact that you have really given blood, guts, and part of your Sunday afternoon, they actually think less of you than they did before they rang for advice on little Willie's snuffles.

They will even spread the message that 'Old doc never minds being called out, he'll go anywhere for a drink'.

Patients never fail to surprise, always asking for new things, making new demands. Only last week a male patient of about thirty-five came into the surgery and said, 'Doctor, could you fix me up with a vivisectomy?' I said, not only was this procedure painful, but there was a society against it. He replied that all his friends were having one, and I said that I was unable to oblige, all I could perhaps help him with was to fix him up with a vasectomy. He went away, smiling.

And, finally, there was a patient who, as part of his medical examination, was asked about the medical history of his family.

78

When asked 'What did your Father die of?' he replied, 'Oh, nothing serious.'

I think patients are marvellous.

Waiting And Patience

'If you can wait and not be tired by waiting,' words penned by Rudyard Kipling as part of the great poem 'If', were not great philosophical thoughts penned after months of deliberation, but his immediate reaction having just queued up to see his doctor.

Waiting is one of the great traditions of medicine. It is much more than just a way of life; in fact it has developed into an art.

Settling Down For A Good Read

A description of some waiting rooms has been given. For the habitual attender just any sort of waiting room is not enough. The quality and variety of magazines is still an important factor and it could be that you might have to sign on with three separate doctors to be sure not to miss any part of a serial in *Woman's Journal.*

The *National Geographical Magazine* makes its last stand anywhere from a ramshackle country surgery to the most modern hospital outpatients; the *Reader's Digest*, with its short, easily read, contributions, is a 'must' for any respectable establishment.

A doctor who neglects the standard of his available reading material will find his list getting smaller, and one who is foolish enough to be indiscriminate and, for example, have too many copies of *Playboy* and *Men Only* available will find his clientele consisting entirely of excited, spotty-faced youths coming for advice about their acne.

Neurotic Fish

Strangely the comfort of chairs, couches, etc. does not seem to be the deciding factor. A good pile of magazines and a wooden bench will always outbid plush armchairs and a goldfish bowl. The goldfish lark has been tried on many occasions, the idea being to lull the patient into a state of tranquillity before his interview. What happens in actual fact is that patients use the tank to wash out their empty bottles or as a receptacle for unwanted medicines, being completely unaffected by the graceful motion of the swimming fish. The result has bred a race of neurotic goldfish who depend on a variety of medicines for their staple food. Also goldfish have now become prone to Farmer's Lung, Housemaid's Knee and similar conditions that had never before penetrated the aquarium.

Keep Waiting

Patients enjoy waiting and, with modern combines and appointment schemes, feel cheated when they are seen almost as soon as they have arrived. Doctors also like patients to have to wait, in order to polish their egos. Although it is said, time and time again, that you cannot measure the practice of medicine in time, because an interview or an appendicectomy can take anything from ten minutes to two hours, most doctors like a good head of patients to have a go at and will usually sit reading the *Financial Times* until their surgery door starts to bulge, when they know there are enough patients to get their teeth into.

Hospital outpatients' departments have carried this even further, and if a doctor is to start seeing patients at, for example, 2 o'clock, the patients will be told to report at 1.30 p.m. The doctor would not dream of starting before 2.30 p.m., and neither would his patients expect him to. A visit to the hospital must be reserved as a full half-day's entertainment. Hospitals are just about geared to the situation, with tea and coffee vending machines, and ladies in green coats selling cakes and sandwiches, whose very existence depends on their having this outlet for their frustrations.

Where To Wait

The patient 'waiting connoisseur' is selective about which surgery or hospital outpatients' clinic he attends. Strangely this is one area of human behaviour where sex on the whole doesn't play a prominent part. It is difficult to feel sexy if your water burns you every time you pass it, especially if you are doing it every five minutes; and diarrhoea, catarrh, persistent vomiting and impetigo are generally reckoned not to produce an aura of romance. However, there are still a few maladjusted men whose selection of waiting place depends on either the shortness of nurses' skirts or the depths of the receptionist's cleavage.

Medical waiting, by and large, has a cosy family atmosphere about it. You don't come back saying, 'I met the most smashing bird at the Doctor's last night'—you are much more likely to say, 'I sat next to the biggest varicose ulcer I've seen', or, 'I have had the most interesting chat with a diabetic who told me that if he pees on the ground all the ants come for miles to inspect his offering. It's the sugar,' he explains.

Class Will Out

These are the main group of patient waiters, the group who come to broaden their knowledge of the various maladies mankind can suffer from. This area of human behaviour is just like any other in that it has different social levels—the more serious the condition, the greater the prestige.

The whole surgery or clinic will be buzzing with anticipation when a new, pale faced, young man drags himself painfully in. But if all he can produce is a boil in an unmentionable place, he will have about as much class standing as a Hindu 'Untouchable'.

On the other hand, a single patient can come in boasting of bronchitis, asthma, heart failure, arthritis, colitis, and at least a dozen operations, all to be recounted, and he will be given the same veneration normally reserved for such personages as the Queen Mother or the Archbishop of Canterbury.

The female patient always has the advantage of having childbirth up her sleeve. Who is in a position to argue if she says she needed thirty stitches after the last one, was in labour for seventy-two hours, and the doctor said her womb was like an old paper bag? Provided she has a new and captive audience there is no romantic length to which she cannot expand herself. This is just one more factor in the uneven battle of the sexes.

The waiting room bore on the other hand has, from time to time, to change doctors, having exhausted the listening potential of a particular Practice list. She moves on to another one, with the added zest to her stories of the malpractices of the last doctor who treated her. 'Straight from Medical School he was, and sent to learn on people like me.'

The Regulars

The final and most interesting group of patient waiters are those who use medical waiting rooms purely as a place for social gatherings. They generally form the hub of what is going on. It is here that you learn who is pregnant by whom, and where she is going to have her abortion. The regulars are like a closed shop. Their only difficulty is thinking up some fresh ailment each week to justify their waiting room place. They are all very concerned about each other and will sympathetically cluck when each one of the closed shop presents his malady of the week.

This group is essential for any thriving general practice because they are able to advise newcomers about the selection of members—'Horses for courses' as you might say. They all treat you as if you were bloody vets anyway. They are all ready to offer advice on diagnosis and treatment and are undisputed experts on character assassination. One mother regular recounted how she had to treat her son for shock. He told her that when his school teacher, who was wearing a low 'V' neck, bent forward, one of her lungs fell out. 'Just shows what happens when these young women start voting for the Liberal Party,' she said.

One regular who was eventually hoist by his own petard, after a great struggle, persuaded the young assistant doctor to give him a card for his wrist (which he thought he had hurt at work) to be x-rayed. With new fields to conquer in the hospital outpatients he became so engrossed in community conversation that he missed his turn for a picture. Not to be outdone, he pushed his way into the x-ray department when they shouted 'Next please'. He didn't know that this was the barium enema queue, and he had two pints of white emulsion paint squirted up his backside before he could say 'Jack Robinson'. What a tale to tell when he got back to the home surgery, and a white tail too.

No surgery would be without this group of people. Whilst they are about the doctor always feels wanted. The only danger they run into, as commonly happens in the fullness of time, is that when they do get something wrong with them, nobody will take any notice.

They have a language terminology of their own—'Devil's Grip', 'Agonies of pain', 'Bronikaltubes', and 'Green colic'. They believe in rubbing-in lotions, ointments and massage. One group member who was also a regular at the local chemist used to call there every Friday night for a contraceptive and a shampoo. We always wondered how he spent his evening.

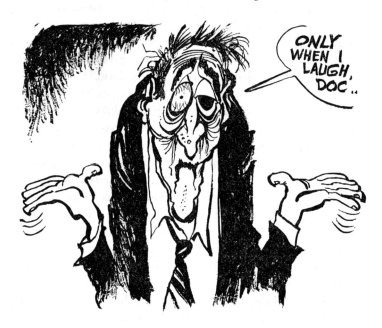

CHAPTER TEN

Patients' Rights

PATIENTS are the most important part of any medical service. They should point out firmly to their doctors, particularly if they feel the doctor is being impertinent, and asking too many personal questions, that patients are doctors' sole source of income. If everybody was well the whole medical profession would be out of work. If your doctor is large and athletic, it is suggested that you do not bring this up when you have called him out in the early hours of the morning to see if he thinks you will be fit enough to attend the Arsenal/Spurs match that afternoon.

On an average each patient visits his doctor four to six times a year. The most infrequent doctor visitors are the people of the West Riding of Yorkshire. Then, as you descend county by county, south and west, the patients' visit-to-the-doctor rate goes up; so Cornwall is worse than Devon, Devon is worse than Somerset, Somerset is worse than Gloucestershire, and so on.

There are two main reasons for this. One, the farther north you get, the greater the number of fish and chip shops there are, and these stay open later, so if it's a choice between a fish and chip shop and the doctor, the shop nearly always wins. Two, there being this increasing tradition of doctor visiting the farther south and west you go, if you are seen by the local populace not to be doing your bit, you are quite likely to be cold shouldered at the Women's Institute, and thrown out of the Buffaloes.

Visiting or being visited by your doctor is of great importance. If, for example, you haven't been able to see your eighty-nine-

year-old mother who lives in the next street for three years, because you have been too busy, ring your doctor on a Saturday
afternoon and insist on him visiting her. You can always say
she is not as well as she was—it's a fair bet. The tears of joy in
your mother's eyes when the doctor tells her you have taken
the trouble to insist on this visit are well worth hearing about;
in fact the doctor will probably call you in himself to tell you
about it. The likelihood is that he will call on her afternoon out
with the Silver Clouds, and will have to leave a note.

As patients, be conscious of your rights. Don't forget you can
sue doctors, report them, write rude words on their cars or ask
them to be the President of your Pigeon Club. They are also quite
useful if you are feeling unwell and wish to feel better again.

Our National Health Service

Also remember that the National Health Service is your own
Service. It is free and, like anything else that is given away,
should be explored/exploited to the very limit.

The average man in the street has four main requisites. He
wants an adequate income, sufficient clothes to wear, furnished
accommodation, and food to keep body and soul together.

Diligent application can wrest all these necessities from the
treasure chests of the National Health Service.

Income. An adequate income for a married couple can be
obtained by them both falling down at work in front of the foreman, writhing on the ground for a couple of minutes (don't
forget to wear old clothes to work this day), then rising, or trying
to rise, clutching their backs. It is not suggested that both husband and wife fall down in front of the same foreman at the
same time. It is better if they work in different places, but if the
Bailiffs are pressing, it is suggested that just the husband falls,
and the wife feels her back go whilst she is trying to lift her
stricken mate off the floor.

Hints on Back Ache

There are many other conditions that one might be presented
with, but other than actually doing harm to yourself, pain in

the back is one of the few conditions that is indisputable. An aid to keeping your back in an unnatural position is to remember, every morning, to do the top button of your vest up to the top button of your underpants, but be warned that if you use this technique for more than a few months, undoing of the button is quite likely to make you fall over backwards.

It is essential that both the tragedies to the husband and wife are entered into the Works' Accident Book, this last effort being the last piece of work that either need necessarily do for years. Both are now assured of a steady income, much larger than they would have if they continued flogging their guts out twelve hours a day. They are assured of this as long as the back disability lasts. The only cure I have ever known for 'chronic back strain' acquired at work was a huge lump-sum settlement for compensation, and a promise of a soft job. This meant that after the lump-sum had been spent at Blackpool, and two full days at the soft job spent supping tea at the Works' canteen catching up on local news, when the victim went for his next fall he had to come up clutching his leg rather than his back, to the murmurs of his late workmates who were saying, 'Poor old Joe, you know he came back to work far too early after that back.'

Set up for Life

If the wife were only doing a two-hour job a week, and paying a 9p stamp, Industrial Injury Benefit should bring her in about £8 to £11 a week, and the husband, depending on how much he has been earning before, would first of all get his income tax back, his sick pay, his Industrial Injury pay, and he would also receive some income from the accident insurance policy he had fortunately taken out a week before the accident, just in case he had an accident. Having established these awards, it is advisable, from then on, to garden at night, because some busybody might report you to the scrutinising officials.

You do not want to spend your hard-earned money on inessentials like food and clothing when there are essentials like cigarettes and beer to be bought.

A Complete Wardrobe

Clothing. Clothing can be acquired under the National Health Service. For the uninformed, the following list should be of great help. Starting at the lowest level, there are plastic anklets, which do help to keep the feet warm in winter. Moving farther afield, elastic stockings, both full-length and below-knee, are always easily obtainable. There are two types, nylon yarn and fine grade, the latter looking fine at cocktail parties. It is a question of getting a prescription and then going to the chemist. You are allowed two pairs of each a year. If they are wearing out go to the busiest surgery a bus ride away and say you are staying there on holiday. This gives the doctor a fee, because you are being treated as a temporary resident. Give an address somewhere in the North of Scotland if you live in London, and if you live in the North of Scotland, a London address.

This applies to all clothing commodities acquired in this way. If you are running out and your doctor won't play any more, go to the next large parish and you can always get a further prescription. Nobody will argue with you, they are too busy with a mass of humanity outside.

Free Knickers

Working upwards, for the nether regions, plastic knickers known as 'incontinence knickers' can be acquired. You probably have to provide a fictitious grandmother who bed-wets before they will hand them over. These are extremely useful, both in wet and dry weather, but tend to get rather hot in the summer. There is a great move to have elastic tights prescribable; until this has actually been passed you have to hunt round until you can find an unscrupulous chemist who will trade them for a prescription for two pairs of elastic stockings.

Moving on upwards again, there are few warmer garments than a surgical corset or, for the more discriminating, an abdominal belt. They are much harder work to acquire, however, because it means not only seeing your own doctor but also being referred to a Specialist. The provident clothes acquirer will make sure that he is seeing two doctors and two Specialists at the same time, thus providing a completer wardrobe. If it does mean more travel to hospital and other districts, you are usually able to get your fares refunded by the National Assistance. As you are in the lowest income group, of course, you don't pay for your prescription and can often do a trade with a working friend by changing the name at the top of his prescription to yours, and charging him half the fee for getting it for nothing.

Do You Need Ear Muffs

Not to be ignored, since it is available, is what is known as a scrotal support. This was specially designed for men with tender feelings, and is usually made of net material, looks like a tea cosy for a goose egg, with an escape hatch at its lower end, and with two long ribbons that tie to each corner. It is ideal as a baby's bonnet, or as ear muffs if you are going ski-ing. It not only keeps your ears warm but, due to the escape hatches, still enables you to hear.

Just a point—if you are going abroad, do make sure that you have sufficient incapacity certificates to cover you whilst out of the country.

There is not much made for the male to cover the chest, unless you are prepared to make armholes in your body belt, fixing the lower end of it with your surgical corset. For women there are, of course, surgical brassiers. These are not only excellent and hard wearing, but by their very construction put inches on your femininity. The individual cups, cut off and surrounded with crêpe paper, make ideal containers for salted peanuts and potato crisps when you are entertaining.

It is actually possible to obtain free alcohol from the National Health Service, but it is so difficult to learn the symptoms of the specific condition that warrants its prescribing that months of training by an expert would be required for you before you were ready. You would probably have to wear restricting garters for three months, with the danger that, even then, you could be whipped into hospital by some know-all and given an arterial graft. Suing the Surgeon afterwards takes too long, and anyway he might really damage you during the operation.

Your Own Personal Loo

The best 20p's worth to be had on the National Health Service is what is known as a 'portable urinal—male'. There is a female one, but it is less efficient and less elaborate. A 'P.U.M.' consists of a complex of tubes, webbing belting and plastic bags, all of which can be detached and used in their own right.

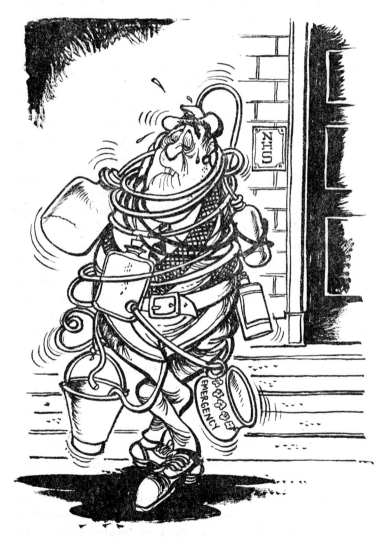

Actually, wearing the appliance can be the basis of a betting fortune, where you can wager you'll drink fourteen pints of beer, then won't go to the toilet for forty-eight hours.

False teeth, glasses, wigs and hearing aids can be acquired through the appropriate channels. If you don't need them, they make very good Christmas presents, and can sometimes be fashioned into ornaments. The hearing aids, if you paint them a different colour and acquire a sufficient stock, will be enough to enable you to go into the mail order business on your own account.

Hernia trusses are not much use to wear. There are two sorts —an elastic truss, or an alternative spring truss which, as its name implies, has a metal band which is always useful. Always ask for a bilateral ingrenal truss. This gives you two pads on a supporting belt which, if hollowed out, make excellent six-gun holders for your sons and their cowboy outfits.

Accommodation. Happily, accommodation is never a problem, just go to the nearest Social Services Office and say you are being evicted (which you probably are) and they will find you accommodation within the next twenty-four hours.

Furnishing. Twelve yards of gauze (which is usually the maximum you can acquire on one prescription) will make curtains for four average sized windows, and incontinent pads (which are 3 ft. squares of paper-covered gamgee tissue) make ideal floor covering. They insulate well, are springy to the foot, and of course are easily replaceable if they get damaged or worn.

Walk In And The Coat Is Yours

This covers basic underwear. The simplest way of acquiring top wearing apparel is to walk nonchalantly into the nearest hospital, if possible carrying a small official-looking black case. Go up to the nearest row of white coats, put one on, walk round with it on for a bit, look at the notice boards, make a few notes in a diary, then walk out. If you do this frequently enough, and the hospital is a large one, you will soon become a familiar face and people will nod to you and expect to see you around. If accosted by a hospital official, speak in broken unintelligible

English, and he will immediately know you are a House Surgeon, and there is every chance that you may be able to have a go at an operation.

The white coats will dye or can be cut up, and can be had in tremendous numbers. Don't overdo this hospital lark. If you are not careful, you'll find that they've put you on the staff, where they will stop some of your money for income tax and National Health insurance.

A Matching Set of Commodes

The much despised commodes are back with us, and unless you are landed with an old-fashioned wooden one, which makes excellent firewood, they are discreet modern chairs with nothing to suggest that the seat lifts off to reveal what looks like a modern aluminium or porcelain cooking pan or casserole with lid. Commodes often have to be acquired through the local Red Cross Society, so be prudent and do not exhaust the stock of your local branch. Six is a reasonable number, and there is every chance that you might get a matching set. You also have the added bonus of the included half-a-dozen containers. If aluminium, as mentioned, they are ideal as pans or cooking dishes, but if porcelain or enamel, which cracks on cooking, are better put aside for use as geranium pots. If, of course, you live in a tent, there is no reason at all why one of these chairs might not be put aside for the function for which it was originally designed.

A trolley pushed out of the hospital while acquiring your white coats will make an ideal mobile bed or dumb waiter, and it is a man of poor ingenuity who cannot turn a few stretchers into bunk beds. You may have to join your local St. John Ambulance Brigade to have access to stretchers. If you do, make sure that they provide uniforms—they are much warmer than the hospital white coats.

Food. Obtaining food on the National Health Service is still a problem. There is always the odd meal in the Doctors' Mess while white-coat acquiring, but the dangers of this have already been pointed out. Since they have stopped orange juice for pregnant mums, it has meant drinking gin neat or with a little water.

A ticket can be obtained for supplementary foodstuffs, but they only give you money, and there is a tendency for this to find its way to the betting shop rather than the supermarket. One can put on shorts and queue for school meals and free milk, but its all rather infra dig and also out of the bounds of the National Health Service.

It is most important to lobby your M.P. about this oversight as there is no doubt it is in this area that the greatest hardships are suffered.

Living off the National Health Service is hard work. It calls for a clear brain, application and ingenuity. It's often much easier to sue your employer for the disability you said you acquired on his premises and get a lump sum—the Union will do all that for you—and then quietly go back to work. You will be in need of a rest.

Among the benefits offered to the general community all categories are catered for, not the least sportsmen, the following short list showing a few of the many benefits available to sportsmen under the all-embracing National Health Service Scheme.

Hernia Trusses for Pogo Stick Jumpers

The ordinary National Health trusses are quite inadequate for the regular pogo jumper, the main difficulty being the tendency of the truss to drop round the ankle of the jumper in mid jump, seriously impeding his progress. There is a standard production truss, but a do-it-yourself home-made kit can easily be fashioned from two bicycle tyre inner tubes. One leg should be threaded through each tube, then the tube looped over the corresponding shoulder. The two now vertical tubes are then joined front and back by simply tying with string then inflating.

This particular appliance is most useful if the pogo jumper wishes to cheat. By inflating the tubes with helium, he can increase leaping potential by twenty feet. It is also useful if you are learning to swim, and by putting your finger over one of the valves on the inflated tube, you can make a rude noise if there is somebody you wish to irritate.

Plaster Boots

These are made to measure boots for patients with broken ankles. To obtain a pair is simple. To simulate broken ankles all one has to do is strap pieces of lead to the lower calf and insist that you keep your socks on when you are x-rayed. This almost guarantees a plaster cast on both feet, enabling you to become an absolute terror on the football field and obtain an unfair advantage in clog dancing competitions.

CHAPTER ELEVEN

Symptoms of Little Known or Hitherto Undiscovered Physical and Mental Conditions

The 'Unt here' Syndrom

This is a condition present mainly in middle-aged Europeans living in Great Britain. It presents as pain, the patient always being able to localise the spot (spots) exactly with a finger while repeating the words 'Here, unt here, unt here'.

Dry Eyeball Disease

This is a condition that affects middle-aged English and American gentlemen who spend afternoons at strip clubs (England), and burlesque shows (America). The eyes, straining to leave their sockets to catch every falling garment or inch of tropical anatomy, in time get so far forward that the eye root gets exposed and becomes dry when in contact with air.

The severe symptoms of this condition can be avoided by either 1. pushing your eyes back with your thumbs before leaving a particular scene of entertainment, or 2. taking a bowl of water into the entertainment with you and immersing your head every thirty-five minutes.

Scrotal Woodworm

Happily, with the new insecticides about, this is a much rarer condition nowadays. The condition arises when, following the removal of one of the two male etceteras, to maintain aesthetic balance, a wooden sphere (prosthesis) is placed in the resulting empty space, thus making the wearer vulnerable to infection whenever he leans against an antique wardrobe or sits on an old chair.

The condition was so prevalent at one time that an alternative material was used—*onyartis picalatis*—i.e. a pickled onion, as described by Professor Tortion, the *B.M.J.* 1919. This appeared initially to be successful until a series of patients complained that every time they kissed their girl friend goodnight they got a yearning for bread and cheese.

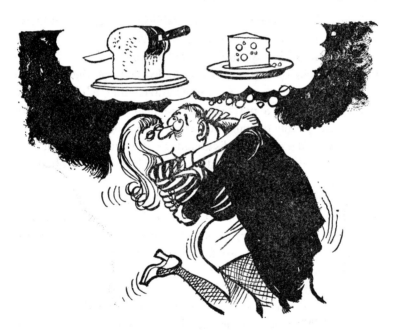

The Ear/Shoulder Disease

It was some years before the cause of this condition was ascertained, the presenting symptom being in both sexes for the patient to appear as if his shoulders were trying to reach up to his ears, or his ears trying to reach down to his shoulders. There was a great deal of research undertaken, and it was only by careful history taking that a final cause was eventually tracked down. The one thing that all the shoulder/ear presentations had in common was that they were stubborn of the bowel, and the shoulder/ear presentation is apparently the maximum position of thrust.

So, if stuck looking for a Christmas, wedding or birthday present for a friend, relative or enemy whose ears look as if they are growing out of their shoulders, remember that a bouquet of senna pods will always be an instant success.

Boiler Makers' Deafness

Boiler Makers' Deafness is an established medical condition. It was found that men working in boilers, exposed to large banging sounds all day, suffer minor hearing damage; the constant repetition of one sound eventually destroys the reception of that particular noise. So, for example, after a certain time boiler-makers have a normal range of hearing except that they cannot hear people banging on boilers. This, on the whole, is an advantage, but can be a disadvantage if your mate bangs on the boiler to draw your attention to the fact it's just about to fall on you.

This particular type of deafness is found in many walks of life. Pub frequenters become unable to hear the word 'Time'. Casanova, the great lover, was at first unable to hear the word 'No' and, later, unable also to hear the word 'Yes'. Husbands lose the faculty of hearing the word 'Money' when their wives are talking to them, and children in epidemic proportions are unable to hear the words 'Wash' and 'Homework'. Politicians suffer most, because in time they become quite unable to hear anything at all said by politicians who belong to political parties other than their own.

There is another similar group who can't hear but aren't deaf—the group who forget to take cotton wool out of their ears.

Tennis Neck

A common disease which occurs mainly in the summer when too much tennis viewing will leave the neck ticking like a metronome long after the patient has come away from the tennis. Tight jumpers and short skirts worn by pedestrian females can also cause a flare up of the condition in male motorists.

Winkers' Disease (always to be spelt with an 'i')

This is caused by an uncontrolled nerve in the eyelid. The owner has no knowledge when his eye is going to twitch. The disease has both advantages and disadvantages. It can result in having your face slapped when you are minding your own business, and your becoming the owner of three prize bulls when you look in at a cattle auction just to see what is going on. On the other hand, the blonde you have been trying to pluck up courage to speak to for weeks might just respond to your flickering eyelid and help you check over the rest of your nervous system just to see if it is working properly.

Frozen Shoulder

This condition has many variations. The main group suffer from a stiffening of the tissues round the shoulder joint, resulting in pain and limitation of movement. It can also be caused by :

(a) keeping your shoulder too long in the refrigerator;
(b) dancing with too many Eskimo women;
(c) walking about nude in the snow;
(d) holding ice cubes under your arm, and
(e) wearing topless dresses.

Splintaris Masticus

This condition occurs mainly in women from the north of England who get splinters in their leaning cushions whilst talking and gossiping over the fence to their next door neighbours. It is a painful condition, and difficult to treat, because it is far too high for Boy Scouts to reach up and remove the splinters.

97

Writers' Cramp

This would seem to be a simple disease, i.e. muscular cramp from writing and holding a pen too much; in fact, by and large, it is a hysterical condition, the hand going into a sort of spasm every time it or its owner doesn't want it to do something, such as writing cheques for Income Tax, shaking hands with Politicians and Trades Union leaders.

I did once mistake it for a form of abuse when, on seeing my aunt off on a Mediterranean cruise, I was splashed by the spray of the large woman standing next to me on the quayside as she shouted 'Writers' Cramp' at a grinning matelot on the upper deck. It was only later that I learnt from a ships' agent that this was Mrs. Cramp encouraging her husband to keep in communication with her while he was on the voyage.

Olecranon bursitis

The name given to the condition where you form small bags of water on your elbows and could really be called Housemaids' Knee of the Elbow. It is caused by constant or intermittent pressure on the elbows. The commonest causes are—

    (a) boozers, leaning on a bar top on their elbows;
    (b) considerate gentlemen lovers who take the weight on
        their elbows.

Thus, a man with a red nose and a right Olecranon bursitis can be easily identified as a boozer, and if your teetotal next door neighbour develops them bilaterally (i.e. on both elbows) suspect that he is having an affair with your wife.

Housemaids' Knee

Housemaids' Knee is the joint halfway between the hip and ankle joint in young ladies who work as maids in houses. It is very similar to Au Pair Girls' Knee but whereas, when a hand is placed on a housemaid's knee it usually results in the knees being brought smartly together, a hand placed on an au pair girl's knee could well bring a verbal response of 'Oh, la la!'

The medical condition of this name is similar to Olecranon bursitis, i.e. constant or intermittent pressure on the knee, causing the formation of sacs of water on either knee.

The commonest cause of pressure on the knee is of course kneeling, and before the advent of household aids such as vacuum cleaners, squeeze mops, etc., the condition was common amongst ladies doing domestic work. However, in this day and age of wonderful gadgets, the highest incidence of this condition is found in Buddhist monks, men who walk habitually on their hands and knees, and crap game players.

Farmers' Lung

Farmers' Lung is one of the two pieces of breathing apparatus that farmers use to breathe with. The medical condition of that name is used to describe when a farmer becomes allergic to his work, i.e. grass, hay, corn dust, and starts wheezing whenever he begins to get busy on the farm. It is a debilitating disease, and usually results in the farmer's early retirement from work. Since the condition was discovered there have been many imitations and, in fact, there are some men who are allergic to all forms of work. I have patients who start itching whenever they start work, irrespective of the type of work, and a small select few who are itching to do any sort of work.

If you can prove that any substance at your place of work causes you to itch, sneeze, wheeze, or come out in a rash, you are made for life and can live happily on industrial compensation (see chapter on Patients' Rights for details). It may of course mean beating yourself with a hairbrush for several weeks until the Company Doctor has definitely ascertained that your undiagnosed rash, which leaves you looking as if you have been beaten by a hairbrush, is the direct result of working for his Company.

Fire Eaters' Throat

This is a common condition amongst circus entertainers who specialise in eating burning objects and spitting out flaming petrol.

It presents with a hoarse or husky voice and is often mistaken for tonsillitis or laryngitis.

With the present increase in the price of fuel, many performers are going in for the lower, cheaper goods, resulting in more frequent carbonisation of the throat and vocal chords. The presenting symptom of this condition is that the entertainer starts backfiring during performances, which is distressing both for himself and his audience. Once diagnosed, the patient is referred to a garage for decoking.

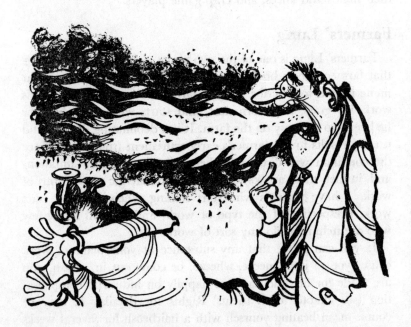

Brush Salesmen's Foot

This condition is used for diagnosing brush salesmen rather than being a medical condition which requires treatment. It is most common in men and presents as disappearing toes on the right-hand foot, caused by having the right foot trapped in doors thirty to forty times a day.

The only way to combat the disease is to change jobs and, if you think you can stand the sex life, become a milkman.

The diagnosis of this condition is most useful in the assessment of character. If, for example, a patient claims he is a publisher's editor, examination of his feet shows that he is suffering from delusions of grandeur and is, in fact, only a brush salesman. If, on further examination, he has callouses on his reproductive organs, then he could be in fact a retired brush salesman who has become a milkman.

Commissionaire's Nose

This condition is most common in commissionaires who stand by revolving doors at their place of work. When the door is situated close to the telephone switchboard, manned by an eighteen-year-old with long legs, black stockings, and heavy upper structures, the distraction caused every time this telephonist bends or leans forward will take the commissionaire's mind off his work and put him in the dangerous position of the revolving door smacking him in the nose. The nose, suffering a constant repetition of this particular blow, will gradually spread over the face and in time no longer be of any use as an air entry into the body.

The commissionaire is then in the position of only being able to breathe through his mouth and is in great danger of swallowing his medals the next time the door gives him a clonk.

Bus Conductor's Pouch

Bus conductors, with the pressure of the standard ticket punching machine, particularly in strong punchers, in time erode the abdominal wall, forming a hollow or indentation directly behind and below the punching machine. This is a natural aid rather than a disease and has the following uses :

(a) To carry your tobacco in if you are a nudist bus conductor.
(b) To keep micro film in if you are a bus conductor attached to MI5.
(c) To keep cigarette ends and ash in if you break all your ashtrays at home.

Its disadvantages are—

(a) When bathing you might get up and find you still had a few pints of water aboard.

(b) When swimming, if your pouch should happen to fill with stones, it might have the effect of causing you to sink.

(c) If you leave your sandwiches in it and forget them for a few days you will become offensive and people won't use your bus; sandwiches last much longer if kept in a refrigerator.

Perhaps the single greatest advantage of bus conductors having developed a pouch is that they become the only group able to ask young kangeroos out for the week-end and make them feel completely at home.

Slimmer's Spot

This only occurs in the most successful type of slimmer; for example, an eighteen-stone man who loses fourteen stone in five days, leaving him in the embarrassing position of having folds of loose skin hanging round his ankles.

The treatment for this situation is, starting at the foot, to work the loose skin up the body to the shoulders and neck and, finally, to the top of the head, where it is all gathered in, taut, and tied round with a piece of string.

Slimmer's Spot is not actually a spot but a change in the position of the navel, in these particular circumstances from the central abdomen area to the middle of the forehead. The male patient thus treated may for some time after his treatment get comments about his crazy tie.

Winkle Picker's Wart

This occurs on the left thumb of avid winkle eaters. On an average a winkle addict eats anything from 7 to 800 winkles a day. To ensure his day's nourishment he has to de-winkle at such a rate that for every eight successful de-winklings he has one miss, where he sticks the pin into his thumb. Thirty or forty years of this constant trauma will cause a raised area of hard, thickened skin to form at the end of his left thumb.

Winkle picker's wart must not be confused with winkle picker's corns which arose on the toes, and were caused by the wearing of a certain type of tight shoes in the 1950's.

Ski Instructor's Zip

This condition is actually a type of pneumonia, in fact a double pneumonia, because it usually affects two people.

With the constant leaning over pupils in the course of the day's instruction, in a certain number of cases, the zip on the front of the ski instructor's anarak will get caught up in the zip on the back of his lady pupil's jumper. The treatment for this situation is to walk in single file (à deux) to the nearest apré ski chalet and be disengaged with wire cutters.

The pneumonia which is the background disease of this condition is caused by the tendency of St. Bernard dogs to rush out and throw buckets of water over the instructor and his pupil on their dual journey back to the chalet.

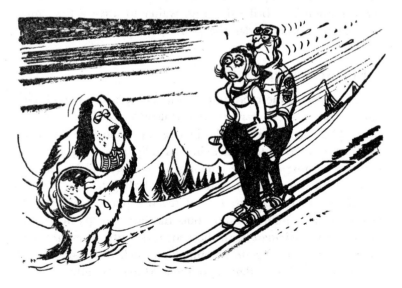

I was able to observe a similar condition occur once in this country when my brother-in-law who was in a theatre party we were attending found that he had entered the place of entertainment unzipped. To hide his confusion he sought to remedy this deficiency by zipping the next time he had to stand up to let other members of the audience pass in front of him. He was almost successful, having reached half zip height, when he realised that he had caught the flimsy dress of the passing theatre-goer in his metal track. I think it was in his memory that placards started to be hung inside gentlemen's conveniences saying 'Please adjust your dress before leaving'.

Alderman's Neck

Alderman's Neck presents as slowly increasing swellings on either side of the neck. It arises from the fact that too many Aldermen have to hang on too long at too many Mayoral dinners, and the bladder being unable to expand past 'Y'-fronts, commerbunds and stiff shirts, sees the daylight round the neck as the only route of escape. It is embarrassing because it leaves a choice between wearing a shirt too big, or risk popping your collar button during the Loyal Toast. The simple treatment for this condition is to bribe the head waiter to leave a few empty champagne bottles under the table within easy reach.

Bank Manager's Lip

This is one of the more unpleasant social/medical conditions, similar in some ways to Boilermaker's Deafness in that Bank Managers, particularly in this day and age of credit squeezes, have to fix their faces in a friendly, reassuring, muscular pattern, pushing out their emotions of horror, delight and embarrassment when they are refusing overdrafts, etc. The constant antagonism of muscle groups and the discipline of keeping the face in a half smiling position puts the lips into spasm, leaving them free to articulate with their tongues, but preventing them from moving their lips to accommodate such essentials as food.

It is a trade secret that most Bank Managers, after a hectic morning, are unable to accommodate their lips to the ordinary cup and have to drink their morning coffee by tipping it into their mouths from saucers. The only way to cope with this situation is for them to chew gum vigorously between customers. However, as most of the larger banking houses are against their Managers chewing gum, many give up banking altogether and often make a good living as ventriloquists.

Barmaid's Chest

This presents as a non-uniformity of the upper works of buxom barmaids. It is caused by the pulling of beer pump handles, resulting in repeated blows to either the left or right hand side of the barmaid's superstructure (depending on whether she is right or left handed). The constant trauma knocks out of shape and upsets the contour of the affected side. For a time metal brassieres were used to alleviate the situation but as on several occasions, flying sparks from nails in the pump handle hitting the metal cup ignited the petrol lighter tube refills on the bar counter, the use of this protective clothing had to be abandoned. The main reason for brewers now pumping most of their beer by compressed air is to reduce the incidence of this condition, and followed pressure from the Barmaids' Union as well as pressure from Union with Barmaids.

Plumber's Joint

This is a painful condition suffered almost exclusively by plumbers. It occurs during the wiping and welding of joints, when the pipe being treated is also at the same time being held by the plumber's left hand. On completing his work the plumber finds that he has welded himself on to part of someone's domestic heating system. Although plumbers often settle well into the households they have become fixed to and can take on small household duties, such as baby sitting and barking in dogless houses that are being burgled, they are left in the vulnerable position of suffering severe burns every time someone fiddles with the thermostat of the hot water system.

Snuff Taker's Eyebrow

Snuff taking is on the upsurge again in Western society and its accompanying medical condition, Snuff Taker's Eyebrow, or 'I am not having him in my house' is being seen more frequently. The taking of snuff requires first the widening (dilation) then retraction (drawing up) of the nostrils, coinciding with the forcing of the eyebrows down on to the upper end of the nose. Constant repetition of this movement will cause the formation of a muscular bridge between the eyebrows and the nose, resulting in a distortion of the face. This is not the great disadvantage it might at first appear to be. It has enabled several sufferers of this condition to be signed up immediately as Martians for the Dr. Who television series. The great disadvantage of the condition is that the eyebrow/nose muscular link results in concerted eye/nose movement. Thus a wink from someone suffering from this condition also produces a simultaneous evacuation of the nose, and there are many circumstances where this is neither aesthetic nor appropriate.

Mental Conditions

Mental conditions come easily to mind. Schizophrenia, paranoid states, introverts, extroverts. Psychiatrists use them as labels to tie on people. On examination each and every one of us qualifies for wearing half-a-dozen labels.

Schizophrenia—split mind

Tell me someone who isn't. Many great moralists read *Men Only* on the side.

Paranoid States—episodes of delusion

Any party political broadcast will give you perfect examples of both suggested paranoia and someone being paranoid.

Introverts

Keep things to themselves.

Extroverts

Shout everything about.
We are all a mixture of both.

Delusions of Grandeur

Who hasn't got them? Some are even impertinent enough to consider they are humorous writers.

Putting mental health in a nutshell, we are in fact all 'Nuts'. If we were not, we wouldn't keep going. Scientists have proved that we only go to sleep to dream. During our dreaming time, we are quietly mad, getting rid of the litter from our minds. If we are deprived of our dreaming time, we become even madder still during the day. It is all a great big joke. We must keep on taking the tablets.

As a medical student I was shown a patient in a mental hospital who claimed he couldn't sleep because he was tuned in to the Light Programme. At the time I laughed, but some years later, on sober reflection, I think that he quite probably was.

Mental illness nomenclature shouldn't be despised. The only comfort that keeps most of us going is that we know our employers/bosses are schizophrenic, paranoid, and have delusions of grandeur; in fact, the only two people I know who are all right are thee and me, except that I am not just too sure about thee.

CHAPTER TWELVE

ABC of Health

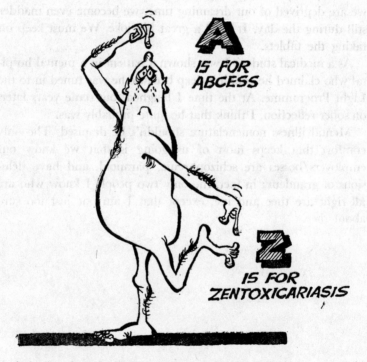

A is for abscess, wherever it may be. A collection of poison coming to a white head—exactly the opinion you have of your immediate superior at work.

B is for baldness—a secondary sex characteristic. Beware of

bald men—they are always randy. Alopecia areata (patchy baldness) is caused by worry. It means you are getting too 'hairyated'.

C is for colon, one of the large intestines, inflammation of which causes an upper class condition known as colitis, which entails spending months at places like Leamington Spa, sipping the waters in the morning and having something unmentionable done to you from behind by a young man with a hose pipe who still calls you Sir in the afternoon.

D is for diarrhoea (intestinal hurry), and some of this country's best runners have not necessarily competed in the Olympic Games.

E is for earache, enteritis and 'eart burn, if you live on the eastern side of London. One of the best ways of making a Maltese cross is to stick your fingers into his inflamed ear. Enteritis is the same as colitis, only higher up. 'Eart burn is a sort of working-class indigestion which occurs most commonly at night after twelve pints of beer, a bowl of peas, some faggots and under-cooked rock salmon in the best batter.

F is for feeding, which we all do, but is chiefly applied to babies in this day and age, who are mostly fed from the bottle, the bottles getting darker and stronger as they get older, many still being bottle fed in their seventies.

This is a pity since it has almost been forgotten that the two ornaments on the front of most women's various sized chests are in actual fact do-it-yourself home milk producing kits. Their product is inexpensive, portable, you don't ever burn a pan whilst you are preparing it, the stuff doesn't go off, and if you don't use them when you have small children, you have to carry them around for the rest of your life as undetachable decorations.

G is for gout, glandular fever, and one of the unmentionable social diseases. Gout is not a disease of the upper class, as you explain to your Irish labourer working on the M1, it is an inborn error of metabolism: what it really means is that a lot of people will have painful big toes. Glandular fever means fever with lots of little round swellings all over your body, and the unmentionable social disease, beginning with 'G', of course can't be mentioned.

H is for hernia. These can be worn all over the body. They appear most commonly in the groins, in the region of the umbilicus, and if you are very clever you can have one inside, which nobody can see, which they call a hiatus hernia. They are the reason for trusses being made which, by exerting pressure, stop them enlarging too much. If untouched they will gradually get bigger and bigger, and the biggest on record is one weighing 173 lb., by a man who lived in India. The only way he could get about was to put it in front of him and push it round in a wheelbarrow.

I is for intussusception. This is a word not known generally to the public, but it is the name given to the procedure when you get a knot in your guts. It results in vomiting and pain, distension, wind and swelling. I hope that the readers of this book will use the wisdom of its pages to increase their social tone and, in future, rather than say 'Get knotted' in the heat of an argument, go and tell their friends to 'have an intussusception'.

J is for jaundice, which means going yellow. This is most commonly caused by gall stones, hepititis, eating carrots, drinking yellow paint, covering yourself with iodine, being Chinese or Japanese, or standing under fluorescent lighting.

K is for kyphoses, and when you call a man kyphotic it means that his spinal column is twisted in one way or another, bending him over. It is not an expression for telling a Welshman called Ky to push off.

L is for laparotomy, which means opening up to have a look. This is when a surgeon is in doubt. The fun is rather being taken out of it nowadays because they have a laparoscope, like a submarine's periscope, which they push through the stomach wall and have a look round. They often find that many a patient's already been torpedoed.

M is for massage, one of the most beneficial forms of medical treatment. It is carried out by ladies in short skirts, called physiotherapists, and when in doubt as to the diagnosis of an emotional condition, you toss a coin—heads they go to the psychiatrist, tails they go to the physiotherapist. All parts of the body can respond to massage, some very much more than others.

N is for nystagmus, of which there are several sorts, the commonest being endemic among coal miners who work in a bad light. It means your eyeballs twitch from side to side. There are several other medical causes, but if you want a clear illustration of the symptoms of this condition you just have to watch the eyes of the men sitting in the front row of the Raymond Revue Bar, Soho.

O is for osteomyelitis or 'ormones if you come from the same place as the man who had 'eart burn. Osteomyelitis is an infection of one or more of the bones, causing heat and inflammation; but if a young lady has hot legs it doesn't mean she is going down with osteomyelitis—it just usually means that nature has endowed her very well in this particular department. 'Ormones, which we all have to some extent or another, are just things that help to make the world go round.

P is for pyorrhea, the condition which your best friend won't tell you about. It does result in inflammation of the gums, and halitosis (bad breath). It is why most of the deodorants are bought. I understand there is a deodorant just marketed, where you swallow a tablet, become invisible, then everyone wonders where the smell is coming from.

Q is for 'Q' fever. This is not the temperature you get waiting outside the Labour Exchange, queuing for a bus, or trying to get in to the local football ground. It is a virus infection, originating in Queensland, Australia, and is transmitted in some way by sheep, so if you have any sheepish close friends, beware they don't give you 'Q' fever.

R is for rheumatism, for which there are many cures, none of which is any good, but include wearing copper bracelets, sitting in churchyards with your fingernails stuffed with peppers, putting your slippers pointing north when you get into bed, eating hot onions with your finger and thumb on your nose, or tying a potato to the end of your bed. The main advantage of this condition is that you usually get two or three hours' notice before it starts to rain.

S is for stones, scabies, and the other unmentionable social disease. Stones can be found in most places of the body—bladder, kidney, gall bladder—and make fine ornaments for the mantelshelf. Scabies is a horrid, antisocial disease, which is on the increase, which you usually get by sharing the same bed-linen with somebody who has previously had it. If you are unfortunate enough to have scabies, the unpleasant social condition beginning with 'S', and the unpleasant social condition beginning with 'G', you then have what is known in the world of gentlemen sailors as 'The Shanghai packet'.

T is for tennis elbow, tetanus and tremors. Tennis elbow is the swelling you get on your left elbow by leaning too long on the bar of public houses; tetanus results in lockjaw, which is the thing you try to wish on your mother-in-law; and tremors are what you get when you've got a tennis elbow through leaning on a bar through trying to keep away from your mother-in-law who hasn't as yet developed lockjaw.

U is for uvula, the little bobble at the back of your throat. Nobody ever explained to me what it's for; ear, nose and throat surgeons sometimes take it out in a temper, one or two people have been able to tame their's and waggle them to order. Otherwise they are of little use except, if tickled, will help to make you sick, which is an advantage or a disadvantage depending on whether you feel you want to be sick or not.

V is for verrucas, which are warts on the sole of the feet that you tread into the feet. Nobody can cure them and, in time, they cure themselves. If you cross a gypsy's palm with silver, you then know that in the next ten to fifteen years they will almost certainly have gone.

W is for writer's (Reiters) Disease. If you have this condition it does not mean you are just about to write a best seller, it is in fact one of the lesser known social diseases like 'S' and 'G', and the only person you should write to is your doctor.

X is for xantho matosis, which means you have an excess of cholestrol in your body, and you start pushing crystals out, both under your arms and in your groin, and in severe cases behind your ears. This is an important part of knowledge to have at the back of your mind because, if you ever find crystals in your girl friend's armpit, you can tell her quite clearly she is coming down with xantho matosis—not to be confused with myxomatosis.

Y is for your own personal malady. May you enjoy it, and may you live happily ever after.

Z is for zentoxicariasis, a new condition which I have invented so as to be able to finish off this alphabet. I have not, as yet, decided what the symptoms of this condition will be, but they will be something that's the absolute end.

CHAPTER THIRTEEN

Television and Medicine

WITHOUT A DOUBT, television has been one of the greatest boons to General Practice. Its reorientation of family life was as if it were designed specifically to help the General Practitioner.

Now, for any late call, be it summer or winter, your patient is nearly always in. Whereas, before, if you didn't go quickly the patient would not wait if the programme at the local cinema started before you had arrived. You used to get so fatigued doing a round of visits at 11.30 p.m., issuing certificates saying that the returning picturegoer was unfit for work the next day, and invariably your stethoscope got 'fish and chippy'.

By carefully studying the *Radio Times* and various regional magazines, if you choose your programme carefully, you are almost 100 per cent sure to catch your patient in.

The front door is thoughtfully left open so that nobody has to come and let you in. You walk to the door from which all the noise is coming, peer into the smoke-filled atmosphere, and if you can catch anybody's attention he will indicate that it is young Elsie, lying on the settee with a bad chest, who is the reason for your call.

Thus the stage is set; mother, father, George, Harry, Joan, Bert, Mary and even Elsie on the settee, all have their eyes glued to the TV set.

You uncover Elsie's chest, trying to disturb her as little as possible, and certainly never obstructing her line of vision. Once you have got your stethoscope on her chest, you are then able to turn and watch the programme yourself, but of course your stethoscope does tend to interfere with the sound. If you have a dual purpose stethoscope, it is much better to use the diaphragm attachment rather than the bell on these occasions.

I prefer ITV to BBC for medical visiting, because sometimes, in the more serious cases, it is possible to take a proper history while the Commercials are on.

Grandma Knows Best

The greatest boon of all is the way it has, with its multiple medical programmes, so fully educated the public. You are now able to discuss the most complicated medical conditions with anyone, even illiterates. The only difficulty is having to explain why grandma can't have an angiogram for Christmas, even if she is entitled to it under the National Health Service, and that making Tommy donate one of his kidneys for research is too big a punishment for coming bottom of the form.

Although few of the general public know how to stop a nosebleed or tie a simple bandage, most are well up on heart transplants, corneal grafts and limb amputations. The specialised branches of medicine also benefit. There is closed circuit television for operations. I have never quite worked this one out, but they say it's good. I believe it means that surgeons are able to watch themselves whilst operating. I once suggested that it would be cheaper and easier to have a nurse holding a mirror; for some strange reason they threw me out of the theatre!

The All Seeing Eye

Television cameras in tubes can now be poked into all sorts of orifices of the body. Nothing is private any more. By swallowing one, the battle between my stomach and the food and drink I threw at it at Christmas can actually be watched and filmed like 'Match of the Day', and a series of horror films is immediately available if one of those all-seeing tubes is pushed up from below rather than down from above.

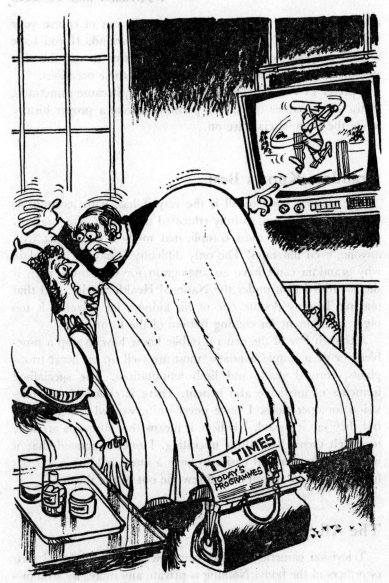

A Birth Between Overs

One glorious summer afternoon, I conducted a confinement in a bedroom where a thoughtful husband had fixed a set at the foot of the bed so that we could watch the England v. Australia

Test. Between pains I lay on the bed next to the wife, criticising the bowling, and during pains crouched at the side of the bed exhorting her to 'try and push it out before the next over'.

In the winter it is great fun watching the course of some particular sport from house to house, seeing how quickly you can go from one visit to the next. My record was during a Rugby International, where I watched the full back placing the ball for a conversion whilst I examined a tonsillitis, then by racing next door saw the same ball flying between the posts while I examined a croup.

A Queue For the Box

All doctors, of whatever branch of medicine, love to appear on television. They sit, looking solemn, pulling their ear lobes, with all sentences punctuated with 'er's'. The reward comes next day when their surgeries and consulting rooms are packed with patients who have come to say, 'I saw you on the telly last night, doctor'. And, whatever the doctor/patient relationship before, even if your particular chap had refused to come out the last five times you called him at night, from now on you are his champion. He must be famous. He has appeared on the 'box'.

This is fine in England where, as yet, they have not used up all the doctors, but in Ireland where there is a very similar TV camera/doctor ratio, each doctor has so far been interviewed at least three times.

A famous English physician, approached by one of the independent companies to appear in their current chat show was told that the programme lasted thirty minutes and the fee was fifty guineas. 'That's fine. I'll pay,' he said.

Somehow other peoples' sets always seem to have better programmes than my own, especially on Sunday afternoon, when my wife won't let me watch, and I may have to spend up to an hour examining an abdomen just to see the film of the week.

A recent survey on the teaching of medical students has proved statistically that they learn much more quickly by watching operations and ward rounds on closed circuit television than they do by actually participating in the operating theatre or attending ward rounds.

There is every chance that, soon, a doctor, if the present trends continue, will be able to qualify without actually ever having seen a patient in the flesh, and more quickly too.

We perhaps will head towards the state where television will become so proficient that, after qualifying, the doctor won't have to see patients in the flesh at all. This can only be for the good, for if your doctor isn't taking the interest in you that you think he should, it is obvious he must have switched over to another channel.

CHAPTER FOURTEEN

Smoking and Medicine

THERE IS a great drive by the medical profession to stop people smoking. It is pointed out as one of the greatest hazards to health, and eminent doctors will go and lecture anywhere about this particular hazard, travelling from lecture hall to lecture hall at 95 miles an hour in their Aston Martins, screaming round corners, knocking pedestrians down like ninepins.

It is put down as the cause of all chest complaints. It is always a great help to find a patient who smokes because at least there is something you can make him give up. If he doesn't smoke you are stuck—there is no direction to point him.

A Respectable Smoke

There is some differentiation between the toxic contents of the various things you smoke, cigarettes being far the worst, pipes and cigars being fairly respectable.

Considering the three conflagrons I personally think that cigarette smoking is a filthy habit and I have little time for those who become addicted to this pernicious weed. For doctors to continue to inhale these carcinogens is a sign of moral ineptitude, knowing full well the dangers to which they are exposing themselves.

Pipe smokers are little better, what with their spitting, tapping and sucking, and the smelly brown tamping finger they all acquire, which must be quite noxious to patients who have to suffer its caress as part of their medical examination.

Some years ago I became an occasional cigar smoker, which has all the advantages over the other two types of oral conflagration.

Cigars, like wines, have a quality of their own, and you can explore the character of each particular brand. I discriminated, and the bigger and more expensive the cigar, the more I enjoyed it.

A cigar smoker carries the air of a man of prosperity and taste. Also there is the added satisfaction of knowing that this type of smoking avoids most of the medical dangers of other types of nicotine intake.

Over the years my appetite for cigars has gradually increased, and although my first choice is Havana, I will smoke anything brown and inflammable. I had great pleasure, whilst on holiday in Spain recently, in smoking a local product which was a foot long, had a green fungus growing on one end and cost the exorbitant sum of twopence.

My Own Smell

I am now as well and truly hooked on cigars as anyone can be hooked on anything. People can smell me a hundred yards off, even when I am not smoking! I am one of the few people who smoke a cigar before breakfast, and the only real strain that has been thrown on my marriage is when I have tried to smoke one in bed. My wife tells me that the sight of a box of Simon Bolivar will bring a gleam into my eye that not even she can produce.

I now smoke as many cigars in the course of a day as a heavy cigarette smoker, though less neoplastic costs me five times as much. I don't usually smoke during the surgery, because my viewing rate is so high, I don't have time to put my hand in my pocket. But, if I have to fill in for a colleague who is sick or on holiday, when time is a little freer, then the room is soon filled with cigar smog and the patient has to grope his way past the 'No Smoking' signs to what must appear to be the Black Hole of Calcutta, and feel his way to a chair.

An Attempt At The Record

One off-duty Sunday I made an attempt on the National Cigar Smoking Record, and including three stops for meals managed to get through twenty-four small ones and three big ones in the course of the day.

My palate has gone to pot—and my tongue is so tender that I am barely able to hold in my mouth the last few cigars of the day. I believe I am even beginning to dissolve the fillings in my teeth.

Once, whilst trying to decide whether the pain in my chest was a cancer of the stomach or a coronary thrombosis, I managed to stop smoking for forty-eight hours, and my symptoms disappeared. There must be some tie up.

When my wife was out the other day I tried one of her filthy cigarettes. It wasn't at all bad, and I find they are only a fifth of the price.

Rats With Hacking Coughs

In the anti-smoking films there are always pictures of encaged mice and rats smoking cigarettes, then terrible pictures of the

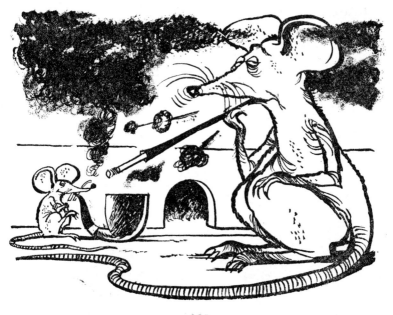

state of their lungs afterwards. In the particular house where I live, we are plagued by both these types of rodent. Yet, in spite of the fact that we purposely leave out a temptingly open box of cigarettes, none is ever taken so either our mice and rats have read the literature or we have colonies of non-smokers.

Most people, frightened into giving up smoking, having enjoyed it for years, become nervous wrecks biting their finger nails, and either commit suicide or have a coronary thrombosis.

It has been proved statistically that heavy smokers in stress executive positions, who give up smoking suddenly, are more likely to die of a coronary thrombosis than they would have been from cancer of the lung if they had kept on smoking.

* * *

In spite of all the Health Officials' efforts, I think smoking is here to stay, though I hope the recounting of my personal experience will be a deterrent to the aspiring smoker.

All who have digested the preceding paragraphs on smoking will have a further insight into their addiction. If they are not cured and require further help, put a blank cheque into a blank envelope. You can always roll it and smoke it if you run out of tobacco.

CHAPTER FIFTEEN

Medicine and Handwriting

WITH THE constant flood of new preparations, new packaging and new type applicators, getting patients to take the right preparation for the right illness and in the right manner becomes increasingly difficult.

As Prescribed By The Doctors?

The man who, when asked how he was getting on with his course of suppositories, replied, 'Not only are they difficult to swallow, but for all the good they do me, I might as well have stuffed them . . .' is now no longer exceptional.

I once found that a patient who was given a sticky paint for tonsillitis, painting the outside of his throat and complaining that he could not get unstuck from his shirt.

Another, having found that antihistamine drops were proving successful in a case of a runny nose in a young girl, I told the parents that it would be a good idea to change to antihistamine tablets, only to find, a week later, that they had been cramming them up her nose.

Commonly, patients have swallowed, or unsuccessfully sucked, the piece of rubber foam packing in the top of tubes of lozenges, and I shudder to think what happens to some of the various sprays.

Even more difficult is persuading patients to take the right preparation for the right condition. When recovering from some malady they tend to give credit to the particular preparations they are taking at that time, irrespective of whether it has any bearing on the case or not. Nor is it always in their best interests to persuade them otherwise.

Probably many great discoveries are made in this way.

It has led to my collecting a series of treatments that always completely baffle my holiday locums.

They include:

● An asthmatic who can only be cured with a stomach bismuth (the green medicine).

● Three people who are sent to sleep with Tabs. Vitamin C, and two woken up by it.

● One man who takes female contraceptive pills to keep his bowels open, and one special lady who swears that it was her new glasses that cured the tenosynovitis in her wrist.

I persuaded a well-known orator friend who used to swallow a mouthful of petroleum jelly before each oration to 'lubricate his vocal cords', that he was wasting his time since the jelly missed his cords by about two inches and went straight into his stomach.

As soon as he stopped, on my advice, his voice became hoarse and rasping every time he spoke.

One beaming patient came in to tell me that they had x-rayed her head to look for her brain and fortunately they hadn't been able to find anything (I believe it, too).

A Cure For Cats

My most famous case was of a man who, visiting his doctor for arthritis, and his vet for his cat's distemper on the same day, got his tablets confused, and now swears there is nothing better than a cat's worming powder for your arthritis, and if you want a sparkling good healthy cat, cadge some arthritis pills from your doctor.

General Practitioners understand that no patients are ever cured unless they have a bottle of medicine. The difficulty is remembering the colour you gave last time; if you are wrong, you can always claim that the new shade is better.

Handwriting

One of the difficulties in prescribing patients' medicines is that they have to be written down by the doctor.

Indications that I might one day take up the practice of medicine as a career came at the age of five and a half with my first school report, which read 'Lundy's handwriting could be improved'.

Since that time my handwriting has deteriorated steadily in spite of all my efforts to improve it. I have now reached the terrible stage where I can hardly read it myself, and letters arrive at the house with the strangest foreign names attributed to the occupier. These are from people who are replying to letters from me, and have tried to interpret my signature at the bottom.

Sleight Of Hand

The illegible writing of the medical profession is not a deliberate effort to prevent patients knowing what they are getting, nor some mystic tradition handed down. It is a habit acquired by trying to do three or four things at the same time and to do them all too quickly. Often, a doctor may be listening to a patient with one ear, answering the telephone with the other, and writing a prescription at the same time. He will start off with every good intention of writing clearly, but in the effort to finish the prescription at the same time the phone call ends, and the patient finishes outlining his symptoms, the last half of the prescription could well end in a blur of squiggles.

Chemists, who are a race of super intelligent men, can usually decipher them, particularly if they know the doctor. But there are hazards.

If you take three substances like Carbitol (a drug for sleeping), Calamel (a purgative), and Calamine (a solution for dabbing on the skin), in prescription writing they look very much the same, and this could result in the patient drinking sun tan lotion to go to sleep, swallowing sleeping capsules to keep his bowels open, and taking a purgative to stop him from itching. Again, in the past this is one of the ways in which great medical discoveries have been made, but it's not to be recommended. In this particular case there is a safeguard. Carbitol has to be prescribed as Caps. Carbitol, Calamine as Lotio Calamine, and Calamel just as Calamel.

One other hazard in prescribing is the printed head at the top of National Health Service prescriptions which reads: Mr./Mrs./Miss underneath each other. The rapid writer can be up a couple or down one as he takes a passing slash with his pen to cross out two of these three, leaving one to indicate who the prescription is actually for. My bad markmanship has resulted in one mother ringing me to say that whilst she had received a pot of cream to rub in her varicose veins, her three-month old baby had a pair of thigh length elastic stockings for his nappy rash. And I had one man who complained that the cups (nipple shields) that I had given him for his ear-ache and the drops (ear drops) for his wife's breast trouble were having no effect.

Deciphering The Squiggles

Illegible prescription writing leads to illegible writing in one's daily visit book, and several times I have raced round the town

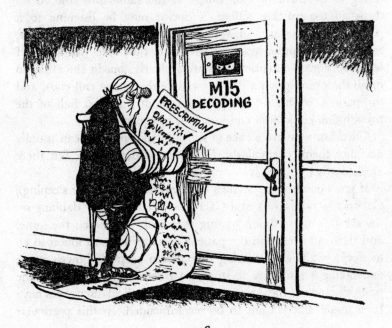

trying to sort out a squiggle at the bottom of my book, and wondering whether it was a missed visit or just a reminder that my wife had asked me to call at the grocer's. Unfortunately, occasionally, by this method of recording, patients do sometimes get missed. My elderly senior partner was once stopped by a woman patient in the street, who said,

'Do you remember me, Dr. Jones?'

'No,' he replied, 'as a matter of fact I can't quite place you.'

'Well,' she replied, 'seventeen years ago you called in to see me when I had tonsillitis, and you told me to stay in bed until you called again.'

With the decreasing number of General Practitioners, and the rapidly expanding population, there is no doubt that prescription writing will get worse and the visiting book will become even more illegible.

There are several answers to this problem. One is to set up writing schools for doctors, but none of them would have time to attend.

The other practical scheme would be to have made up rubber stamps of all the prescriptions, so that the harassed G.P. can just dab on to his pad the drug of his choice.

It would, however, be essential for somebody to have written legibly on the handle of each rubber stamp what it was actually stamping. Clearly no doctor could do it.

CHAPTER SIXTEEN

Hospitals

HOSPITALS VARY from massive steel and concrete pseudo Hiltons, with private rooms and piped television per bed in the United States to three-in-a-bed wooden shacks in Africa, with the family roughing it outside and cooking your food.

The principal reasons for hospitals is to carry out medical treatment and investigations that cannot be carried out in the home. It was commonplace at one time to have your appendix and tonsils out on the kitchen table. The pendulum has now swung so far the other way that not even Howard Hughes could get his hip operated on on the top floor of the Dorchester Hotel.

To many, hospitals are homes of rest, and the only place where you don't have to get your own meals ready, and for some the only place where the roof doesn't leak. Unless, of course, you are in the wooden hut three-in-a-bed situation, where you are never quite sure if the damp bed is due to the roof or one of your two bedmates.

The Hospital 'Lifers'

A determined band of people spend most of their lives flitting from one hospital to another. These are the professionals, their peak effort being for Christmas. The real professional is never without food and board. All he has to do is to learn to dislocate something, grow a kidney stone and never let anybody operate on it, or make sure a bone that is broken never heals. If he can show something on x-ray, even if it's only a piece of tinfoil on the inside of his shirt, hospitals are always open. It's much more important to have a positive investigation than it is for anybody to take any notice of what you are saying. It is important, if on the circuit, not to visit the same hospital too often, because you may be recognised and turned out, even if you actually are in pain.

If you start in Cornwall, then steadily work your way up the left-hand side of England, going from hospital to hospital, and coming down the right-hand side when you have finished the left, this is enough to keep you going for some years without even touching the middle. A tip for the beginner—a teaspoonful of sugar in your urine specimen is always good for another week. If you are good at making tea and emptying bedpans, you have every chance they will keep you on the team.

Hospitals are essential. We cannot have enough of them. At some time most of us will visit one, so this book, like all branches of medicine, apart from what curative therapy it offers, also offers reassurance and comfort.

Many people have a great fear of hospital admission and hospital treatment. Notes from the diaries of J. J. Rolls, Esq., Managing Director and owner of the Fenwick Motor Car Company, will, in the finest tradition, be of help and comfort to all people entering hospital.

For some reason he wrote this in his own blood; perhaps they wouldn't allow him ink in the ward. I never knew the outcome of this story, but I do see there is a vacancy on the Board.

Memoirs of J. J. Rolls, Esq., Managing Director of Fenwick Motors, dated the 22nd of February, 1965.

I had picked out the spot where I wished to be taken if I were ever ill. It was a cottage high on the cliff overlooking the sea, with the most magnificent view. That my friend who owns it is a Cordon Bleu cook is just by the way. I know there is a plug for the TV in the room because I have seen it. In the tender balm of these surroundings, although perhaps I wouldn't be in too great a hurry to get well, I would without a doubt thoroughly enjoy the particular malady I was suffering from.

The last place I ever wanted to be ill in was a hospital, as the experience of friends had convinced me that the whole hospital routine is designed not only to prevent you from enjoying your illness, but by applying such a vigorous routine you are actually trying to get better quickly to get back at last to your home comforts.

Fortune would have it that being unwell, after some investigations I was ordered into hospital. I have few indulgences, but I do like a Havana cigar before breakfast; it settles me and I can start the day tranquil and relaxed.

A Cigar Before Breakfast

But on my first morning, lighting my expensive dummy with my morning tea which they had insisted on bringing at 5.30 a.m., had the same effect as letting off an incendiary bomb. Sisters and nurses rushed with fire extinguishers from all directions, and my poor cigar was snatched from my mouth. I was deprived of this necessity for a whole two weeks just because the man in the next bed was in an oxygen tent—and ugh! Tea at 5.30 a.m. The only time previously I had had tea at this hour was when I was driving all day to the Motor Show, and then I had to spend two days in bed afterwards recovering.

I thought there must be some exciting reason for having been got up so early, but the next thing was at six o'clock when they brought round chipped enamel bowls to wash and shave in, and a red coloured liquid to gargle with. By now I did see a little reason in their madness. Here was I at six in the morning, washed, shaved, sharpened by being deprived of my cigar, but really on my toes, hungry and raring to go.

There seemed little action after the wash, so calling the least belligerent-looking staff nurse over, I enquired of the form.

'Oh,' she said, 'you can now go to sleep till breakfast at eight.'

Sleep now? This was obviously some form of subtle brainwashing. They could waken me during the night, wash me, whet my appetite with a cup of tea, and then tell me to go to sleep again.

With my gastric juices now welling in my throat, I managed to pass the next two hours frantically doing crossword puzzles of the two evening papers I had brought with me.

No Bacon For Him

At eight o'clock, with a bustle and change of staff, in came breakfast on a steaming metal trolley. Porridge (which I hadn't had since I was at school, but which now I wouldn't have swopped for caviare) and sausages and bacon. I watched the trolley come slowly down the ward, and I have never seen two little blackened objects and a slab of bacon look so delicious. The trolley seemed to take years as it crept towards me, but at last it did reach me and a plate of this tempting repast was put in front of me. As I reached forward to take my first mouthful, the tray was suddenly whipped from me by a greyhaired sister who was followed by a nurse carrying a sinister looking metal tray.

'No breakfast for you,' she snapped, 'you're for gastric test meal.'

The nurse dropped the metal tray in the place of my breakfast one, and quick as a flash started to push a rubber tube up my nose, shouting 'swallow'.

It was at this stage that I decided even if I dropped dead on the way out, from now on I was going to get better quickly. She kept pushing this endless tube up my nose and wasn't satisfied until I had swallowed two yards of it. 'What about breakfast?' I croaked.

'You have a glass of glucose water at nine a.m.,' she replied, and whisked away.

I like a glass of brandy in the evening. I always enjoy a cup of coffee, and nobody appreciates a glass of wine with a meal more than I do, but a glass of glucose water at nine a.m. is no substitute for any of these.

For the rest of the morning, at hourly intervals, people kept coming and sucking up the contents of my stomach through the tube in my nose and taking it away in bottles.

The Stomach's Ghastly Secrets

This was a gross invasion of my privacy. I have always got on well with my stomach—I have never enquired what it did, and my stomach in its turn never bothered what I did unless the mixture that I threw into it was too rich, when it has protested in its own unmistakable way. Now its ghastly secrets were being exposed in front of me in bottles. It was all so unfair.

All morning, during my hourly syphonings, my own distraction was the ward traffic, which was a close second to Piccadilly Circus. Trolleys coming and going, men waving to their chums as they went off to have their hernias and appendix done, like men leaving for the front-line, returning an hour later, ashen and unconscious, as if they had been victims of the first poisonous gas attack.

Half A Day Gone and No Food

By three o'clock, when visitors came, tired through lack of sleep, weak with hunger, I thought I had been in hospital for three months. By the attitude of my friends, the firm squeeze of the shoulder without speaking and the way they ate my grapes (they will be no use to him), I knew I must have looked pretty ill. Eventually they went and, looking at my watch, I saw it was now four p.m. As I usually go to bed at twelve, there were still eight hours of the day left.

They removed my tubes and at 4.30 I was given some tea and a piece of cake. Things had begun to improve. I felt the surge of strength with my nutrient and began to take a more active interest in what was going on. I did my hair and took stock of the nurses. Gosh! That blonde one would grace any party. I could just imagine her in a low cut evening dress.

I spent the next hour trying to catch her eye. She was obviously playing hard to get. But at last she came smiling towards me, with a little black book in her hand. Boy, what a figure! She was obviously going to date me. A beautiful smile crept across her face, she opened her book and said,

'Tell me, have you opened your bowels to-day?'

This was the end.

I slowly put on my dressing gown, shuffled to the men's toilet, out through the back of the toilet door, down the fire-escape, and away.

Hospital Visitors

This chapter would not be complete without mention of hospital visitors. These are dedicated people who make regular visits to hospitals, talking, and bringing gifts to patients who have no visitors of their own. The vast majority of them are excellent people, doing excellent work, but the few bible-thumping do-gooders who are just filling their own ego can be hard to swallow for both patient and ward staff. One of the worst of this ilk rushed into a medical ward one day, delighted to find the first Chinese patient the hospital had admitted, in an oxygen tent, with no visitors. Full of good works and good thoughts, he rushed to the bedside, offered him a sweet, asked him how he was, and the Chinese seaman looked up and said 'Chang fu, fu chang, chang woo', turned on his side, and dropped dead. Conscientious about his duty, the visitor went to the Chinese Embassy to inform them about the death of one of their subjects. They already had this information, and the visitor, wanting to pass on the patient's last message, asked for a translation of 'Chang fu, fu chang, chang woo', and the Embassy official replied, 'That is easy, Sir, the translation into English is, you are standing on my oxygen tube.'

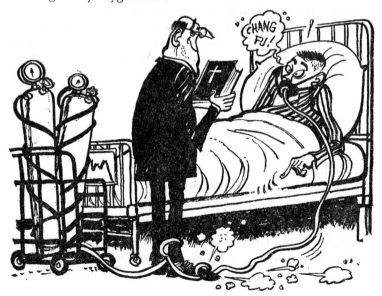

CHAPTER SEVENTEEN

Concise Human Anatomy

The Human Body

The human body consists of a bag of skin enclosing a network of tubes and pipes, the whole structure being stiffened by a framework of bones.

If the outer skin covering is punctured, the contents of the tubes and pipes, principally blood, will leak out. If they do so in sufficient quantities, the body in question will be unable to function.

If one of the stiffened bones is broken, the part stiffened by the bone tends to become floppy and useless to the body.

Parts of the body are detachable without causing too much disability, and some are replaceable, but although great strides are being made in the furnishing of body spare parts, no complete kit is yet available.

The body, in some departments of its more essential structures, carries a fair depth of reserves. For example, the standard body has two lungs and two kidneys, but can function quite well on one-third of this equipment.

The body has remarkable regenerative properties; small holes in the skin will close up, sealing off the leak if the edges are brought together. Blood leaking through broken pipes will stop if the end of the pipes are tied off and the blood will reach its original destination by some other route. Broken bones will join up again if kept still for a time. One of course aims to have the bones join at the same angle they were before they were broken, rather than letting them join crookedly.

The Head

The head consists of a bony shell covered with skin, and sometimes hair, its inner cavity being filled with either brain or more bone. The quantities of each of these two substances can often be accurately ascertained by seeing the particular type of work the participant is doing. For example, it is likely that the political leader of the country would have a higher proportion of brain to bone in his head than would a trench-digging labourer on the M1. Or is it? There are no hard and fast rules and the only positive way of telling is to open the skull and look inside—this unfortunately may be an irreversible process.

The head is usually situated in the mid-line at a variable distance above or below a straight line adjoining the two shoulders. Types of work and play may decide to some extent the position and posture of the head.

Whilst male opera singers and basket-ball players usually have their heads mounted on the top of swanlike necks, there is sometimes, in front-row Rugby forwards and brick-hod carriers, no line of cleavage between the neck and trunk at all.

Soccer centre forwards and fish porters tend to look at you sideways, not because they are of sinister disposition, but because they get into special neck and head attitudes in the course of their work.

Appendages To The Head

As a rule, most heads have a set of standard fittings. These usually consist of two eyes on the upper front part of the head, which may be so close together as to almost touch, or so far apart as to be in opposite corners.

The nose projects forward, usually starting below the eyes and finishing above the mouth. It has been known to start between the eyes and descend to almost cover the mouth.

In sports such as boxing, contrary to the usual projection

forward, a nose which has been subject to constant pressures will actually have been pushed back to fall flat in the face line. At this stage the nose is usually rejected as an organ of respiration.

The mouth is a hole going into the head, usually situated below the nose. It is the main entrance for air entering the body and main exit for swear words leaving the body. It may or may not be lined with teeth.

The ears, or hearing trumpets, surround the hearing canal, and can be any shape or size, and situated virtually anywhere on the head, although it is unusual for them to be situated on the front of the face in the region of the eyes, nose or mouth.

Some people can actually bring air into the body through their ears. This is usually associated with previous injuries to ear drums. I once saved the life of a man who boasted loudly of this talent. His friends had got so fed up with hearing his boasting, that at the end of a drunken party, they held his head under a bucket of water with only one ear protruding, and were chanting, 'Breathe, you bugger, breathe'.

The ears, eyes, nose and teeth can become detached from the head. But, whereas the ears and nose can sometimes be replaced or stuck on again, the eyes cannot be, unless they are replaced by glass replicas, which are of little or no use for seeing with.

For the worker, this has few problems, as he can claim great quantities of compensation from somebody and attribute it directly to his work, although he may have incurred the injury while on holiday at the Costa Brava.

The loss of ears and disfigurements of the nose do not usually affect the life span of the afflicted person, but may add to or more usually detract from his aesthetic appearance.

The Neck

The neck is a cylindrical structure between the head and shoulders, of varying lengths. To stop it flopping about it has a piece of bone that runs down the middle of the back of it, which, if broken, will cease to stop it flopping about.

It is an essential structure in that, although possessing few functions of its own, it connects the head to the body and through it passes air to the lungs, food to the stomach and messages down the spinal column from the brain to the rest of the body, telling where and when and in what way to function.

The disruption of any of these three services can obviously cause great upset to the rest of the body.

As explained in the section on The Head, the presence of a neck in some men is not always at first obvious. Whatever the position of the head, however, the presence of a neck (even if only in rudimentary form) can always be demonstrated by x-rays.

Various manoeuvres with the neck can easily interrupt the three vital services which pass through it.

A tourniquet round the neck will always, and fairly quickly, stop any bleeding above it, but, if left on for more than a few minutes, does put the rest of the body in a state of ill health, as it completely cuts off the three vital services.

There are many different types of neck. Long ones, short ones, fat ones, thin ones, hairy ones, and, perhaps most commonly, scraggy ones.

Apart from the passage of vital services, the neck has many other practical uses. It is ideal to hang things on, but not the best thing to hang from itself. Collars can be buttoned round it, making it more difficult to pull shirts or vests off downwards. Weights in conjunction with the shoulders can be carried on it and in the countries which still practise slavery a yoke can be put round it, enabling the wearer to provide the traction for ploughing.

If the usual air holes for entry into the body, i.e. mouth, nose and ears, are bunged up, a hole in the neck will allow breathing to continue. This is called a tracheotomy. It is sometimes a standard fitting in racehorses. Games players may return to the field and play when it has been done, but are best advised to leave the field actually to have the manoeuvre carried out. It is not the ideal condition to have for making a claim for compensation as it usually prevents you from speaking, so before considering having this procedure carried out, make sure that your Union's representative is more articulate than you are.

Appendages to the Neck

The neck, unlike the head, has no recognised set of fittings. It is, however, a common site for moles, warts, birthmarks, pouches, boils and carbuncles, all of which are detachable, not all of which are replaceable.

In my own experience it has always been wise to try and avoid detaching a boil or carbuncle from another man's neck, particularly accidentally during the playing of a robust physical game or at a party, because it seems to cause extreme activity of the mouth and hands, and in the more ungentlemanly, movements of the feet as well.

The neck itself is not detachable. In cases where this has unwittingly happened it means the immediate cessation of work or, during a team game, the player having to leave the field and take no further part in that particular contest.

A large lump on the lower front side of the neck may mean that the patient has an enlarged thyroid gland. It is wise not to interfere with this as people with increased thyroid activity are often very bad tempered.

The Thorax

The thorax, or chest, is a round barrel-like structure situated below the neck. It has no rigid line of demarcation from the abdomen, but can be roughly said to go down as far as the bottom of the rib cage, with the navel (or umbilicus) hovering below it like a full stop.

It is of special significance in this modern age, because, with the excessive growing of head hair by both sexes, it is left to the thorax to present the actual evidence of differentiation between the male and female sex.

Whereas in most males the surface of the thorax is fairly uniform, apart from scattered patches of hair, in the female there are usually two soft round swellings on the front of the thorax. These are of variable size, shape, position and resilience.

The thorax contains some extremely important organs, viz., the lungs, heart and gullet, and part or all of the stomach. All these organs must work efficiently and constantly for the body to function as a whole.

The thorax is surrounded by a body cage called the ribs, which resembles a series of thick wire fencing attached to the spine at the back and the sternum, or breast bone, at the front.

There are usually twelve ribs and although it has been placed on record that at least one woman has been made out of the fifth rib of a man, this is not a proven procedure, and it is not your first line of action when short of a date for Saturday night.

The thorax is airtight, as it is covered with skin, and the chest is filled by air lifting the ribs up by muscles, thus increasing the space inside, causing a fall of pressure inside the thorax. If the mouth and nose are not sealed off, air will be sucked in through these holes, filling the lungs that are under the same negative pressure.

A leak anywhere in the thorax, i.e. a hole made by a rusty nail or carelessly slung pick-hook, will of course let in more air, thus spoiling the whole sequence of movements, as well as making the victim extremely short of breath.

As a good general principle, it is important to avoid getting holes in your thorax. If for some reason this is unavoidable, either by the nature of your work (i.e. if you are a hatchet thrower's assistant, or a dartboard attendant), do always keep some simple patching material in your pocket to close the hole as soon as possible.

For objects that pass right through the wall of the thorax and stay inside the chest, do seek some help, because (a) they tend to rattle about when you walk, and (b) if you are going to sue whoever was responsible for whatever object entered your thorax, you will need whatever it was as evidence.

The inner lower surface of the thorax is bounded by the diaphragm, which is similar to a polythene sheet with a few holes in it to let some of the more important structures pass through into the abdomen.

The Diaphragm

Like the rib cage, this is one of the participants in making the cavity of the thorax larger in respiration. Whereas the ribs move upwards and outwards, the diaphragm moves downwards. This is important, because, should you have two people sitting on your chest, you will have difficulty in expanding your rib cage, and will have to use your diaphragm breathing. It is never a good idea to have two people sitting on your chest for too long until you know exactly how strong your diaphragm is.

Ribs

Ribs can be broken very easily, and the pain is often not so much in the fracture site—if you are a true hairy man and your injured chest is strapped with adhesive tape without shaving it, the major torment will come when the strapping is removed.

I saw one hairy sailor chase the Casualty Officer of the local hospital round three wards, blood streaming from his chest, and waving a piece of strapping on one side of which hair had grown like mustard and cress in a saucer, and on the other side a thick layer of chesty meat, thus disproving once and for all that comforting medical phrase 'It won't hurt if I do it quickly'.

Broken ribs, apart from being painful, are not usually troublesome unless one end sticks into something vital inside the thorax, e.g. the heart or lung; and if someone presents you with a squashed looking chest, and he is not breathing, always be suspicious of some damage inside.

Strange congenital chest shapes can be confusing. The first case I tried mouth-to-mouth resuscitation on was a tall thin man with a pigeon chest who was holding his breath to try and cure his hiccoughs and was, in fact, only accompanying to the hospital a nephew who had cut his finger.

Another main structure of the thorax is the sternum, or breast bone, which is a favourite site for tattooing, being fairly flat and stable enough for the tattooist to rest his elbow on. It does little else but hold the ribs together at the front, like a billiard cue rest. At its bottom end is a firm piece of gristle, called xiphisternum, which you can wobble about. People are always discovering this little lump while in the bath, and rushing off to the doctors, convinced they have some dreadful growth.

On the back of the thorax are the shoulder blades and the

dorsal spine column which runs down the middle, separating them, and into which the other end of the ribs are fixed.

Nothing very exciting happens to the shoulder blades, although you can of course break your spine in any part.

A shoulder blade detached from the body could serve as a table tennis bat or as a children's spade at the seaside.

On the top of the thorax on either side of the neck are the collar bones, which really seem to be put there to see how often they can be broken by steeplechase jockeys. This is some sort of secret jockey cult, as you never hear who is the champion for the year, or who holds the record for the most fractures.

Appendages To The Thorax

The thorax has few appendages. The notable ones are the nipples, which are usually black spots, but are sometimes brown or pink and have been known to be yellow, indigo and violet, situated roughly in the middle of each side of the front of the thorax. These are usually two in number, but there can be several in a line directly below each main nipple, going as far down

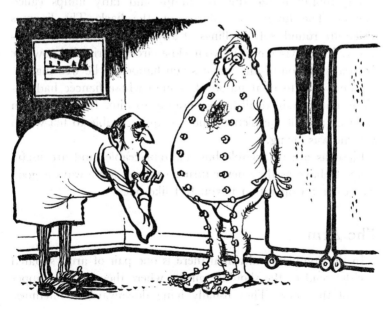

as the groin. These are known as accessory nipples and are remnants of primitive physiological mechanism, in this case reptilian. Quite what this means nobody has explained, but it is comforting to know you are carrying a few spares.

In the female, the nipple surmounts and is the mouthpiece of the standard built-in feeding device of the normal do-it-yourself home childbearing kit. In the male it has little or no use other than as a landmark.

Nipples are always on the front side of the thorax and point (unless he is walking backwards) in the direction the wearer is going. If a neck and head have been rotated round too vigorously the situation of the nipples will indicate which way the face should be pointing.

In the hairy male they will be completely hidden and a fair amount of harvesting may have to be done before they can be located as direction finders.

Nipples are both detachable and replaceable. It is not advisable to go round detaching them either at work or during rough games, because (a) the wearers become extremely annoyed, and (b) they are of little use on their own.

The thorax is the site for humps and fatty lumps called lipomas. The humps are always on the back. The lipomas which are round, soft swellings of any size, can be almost anywhere. It is advisable to let your close circle of friends know the size and situation of any lipomas you happen to be wearing.

I once had to treat for shock a man whose fiancée had unwisely not explained all her geography to him. In the dark, in the back row of the pictures, he was quite unable to tell which way she was facing.

Lipomas are detachable but not replaceable, and are useful lumps to have as they never turn nasty and are always a good excuse for an operation if you feel like one.

The Arm

In the complete individual there is one pair of arms situated at either end of the shoulder girdle, where they join the upper part of the chest. They usually hang downwards. Sometimes, after certain injuries and in at least one psychiatric condition, they point permanently upwards. Their length and shape will give some idea as to the occupation or relaxation of the bearer. For example, whereas members of the Oxford and Cambridge Boat Race crews have one arm longer than the other, depending on which side of the boat they are dipping their oar in, the arms of men who spend too much time wheeling heavy wheelbarrows may hang down to almost touch the floor.

Most arms have a hinge joint in them, roughly about the middle. Its position may vary from an area just below the arm-pit to so far down that there is some difficulty in distinguishing between it and the wrist joint.

The middle or hinge joint of the arm is called the elbow. It is usually a simple hinge; the presence of a soft ball-like swelling on the back of the joint (Olecranon Bursa to the crossword puzzlers) will indicate this arm has been used for leaning on hostelry bar counters and that the wearer uses his other arm to drink beer with. This would appear to be a most valuable piece of information, but as yet I have not been able to find a use for it.

The arm, like the neck, carries blood, nerves, etc. down to the hand under its skin covering, and again any treatment to injuries of the arm which interferes with the supplies going down it will not only prevent the left hand knowing what the right hand is doing, but will leave the right hand in some doubt also.

Tourniquets should not be applied too long to any limb because after about twenty minutes there will be a complete disruption of all services below them.

If you should suddenly lose the services of a hand when you are either:

(a) hoisting a bucket of cement up ten floors by a rope over a pulley, watched by thirty admiring workmates, or

(b) being the middle man in a rope of three climbers, or even

(c) being in the final of the table-tennis championship

there is no doubt that confusion would arise.

The upper arm is stiffened by a bone called the humerus,

although I have never been able to see anything funny about it. It has a round knob at one side of the top or upper end, which fits into the shoulder joint, in what is known as a 'ball and socket joint'.

The ball can sometimes slip out of its socket, thus giving rise to the condition known as 'dislocated shoulder', making the two shoulders look uneven. Not even a Doctor of Theology can tell whether the ball bit of the humerus has been broken off and it is a fractured shoulder joint, unless the shoulder is x-rayed.

A Most Useful Bone

The humerus itself, when detached from the body and surrounding flesh, etc., is a most useful object. It makes an ideal junior golf or hockey club, is the right weight and size for a shillelagh, and can, if you remove the bone marrow and make a hole in both ends, serve as a two-handed church warden pipe.

The lower arm is stiffened with two smaller bones lying side by side, called the radius and ulna. These are not nearly as exciting as the humerus, break very easily and confuse you, and you can break one without de-stiffening the arm. If you break both, the arm does tend to look crooked and loses its stiffness. Pain usually accompanies this process of breaking.

In younger people, the bones will bend without breaking and are given a special name of a 'greenstick fracture' and, even though they are only bent, it hurts just as much to try and straighten them as if they were broken in half.

The radius and ulna, being small, have not the same nor the variety of uses as the humerus when isolated from the body. The radius, as it has a notch in one end, can be converted into a spoon if you are ever wrecked on a desert island. The pair of bones together make passable chop-sticks, and either will beat a kettle drum quite adequately.

Between the lower end of the radius and ulna and the hand is the wrist. Through the wrist pass two main arteries, several important nerves, and in it lie a lot of small bones called carpal bones, each with a funny name.

This is of great importance to doctors, because if you should break one of the small bones of the wrist, they can discourse for hours, using such names as schaphoid, lunate, pisiform, and take repeated x-rays. That the treatment of them all is exactly the same seems to have no bearing on the subject. When detached from the body, the carpal or wrist bones are the right number and shape for playing the old fashioned game of 'stones', and are also extremely useful as standard ammunition for small boys' catapults.

Below the wrists are the hands, which are most useful for carrying things, shuffling cards, blowing your nose, and other small toilet requisites.

A Stitch in Time

The arms, or the upper limbs, as a whole, are most useful. They can become detached with the hairier games and the hairier types of work. Happily it has been discovered in America that they are replaceable, and a detached arm has been stitched back again to function nearly normally.

This work, however, is only in its infancy, and the reader is warned to think carefully before putting himself in the position where one or both of his arms are likely to become detached. If, inadvertently, you should have one arm detached, you must remove yourself immediately from that situation, for to have both arms detached is a considerable inconvenience.

Appendages To The Arm

Most upper limbs have five appendages, viz., thumb and four fingers. It is not uncommon to be born with more than this number and it is quite common to have less, because fingers and thumbs are the most easily detachable parts of the body.

The easiest way to detach a digit is at work with a circular saw, and at games by a bit of old-fashioned biting.

One gipsy tribe insist at their wedding ceremonies that the groom bites off part of the little finger of the bride before the wedding ceremony is complete. It is certainly a discouragement to getting married more than three or four times.

Fingers and thumbs are almost indispensable—they have innumerable uses. They will poke in, up, or around anything. If they have nails on, they can be used to pick coins out of slot machines, and what is most important, to scratch with. They are great aids to counting, and there is no doubt that the 'V' sign made by sticking up the first two fingers in the shape of a V, raised public morale to such a pitch that it certainly shortened the course of the last war. This same sign, with the back of the fingers facing forward, has shortened many a conversation.

Fingers can be used to beckon and point with, and a jab in the eye with a stiffened finger can cause extreme discomfort.

Thumbs-up speaks for itself as a message of good cheer, and thumbs down, in years gone by, meant that a few hungry lions were going to have a Christian indigestion.

The absence of thumbs could have prevented generations of young people hitch-hiking all over the world.

The fingers are stiffened by joint bones called 'phalanges', and are occasionally webbed.The lucky owner of webbed fingers has a decided advantage in school swimming sports or if he wants to make a blowing noise with his hands.

Detached fingers are sometimes replaceable, but having one or two missing causes so little inconvenience it is usually hardly worth the bother. Nowadays if you should lose them all, or even your hand, there are many mechanical contrivances with which they can be replaced. These have the added advantage of stopping you biting your nails and preventing you ever having chilblains on your fingers.

Anatomy Of The Leg

Since the advent of the short skirt the detailed anatomy of the leg has become more obvious and available than previously.

With skirts seeming to stop just below the neck and legs of various shape disappearing up into them, one would expect, on seeing a disrobed victim of this type, to find the legs fixed to the shoulder girdle with only the head above. This is not so. The legs are separated from the head by the abdomen and thorax, without which the female sex would have no base to anchor all their various bits of supporting clothing. There is often so much support in so small an area that medical cases presenting as shortness of breath, hump back, swollen legs, purple face, can sometimes be cured in a few minutes by the simple operation of undoing three vital buttons or one zip.

The legs, which are two in number, are joined to the outer lower corners of the abdomen by another ball and socket joint. Unlike the shoulder, the ball of the leg bone (femur) which fits into the socket (acetabulum) of the pelvis, is on the end of a short bone joined at right angles to the femur and is called the femoral neck. There seems to be no benefit in this, other than that the short bit of bone breaks very easily (fractured neck of femur) and is mended by having a nail driven down it. This is a great boon to the medical profession since it is the first bit of the body they have learned to nail back successfully, and you are able to walk on your leg a week after you have broken it.

The femur, or bone of the upper leg, is a similar, larger shape to the humerus of the upper arm, and like the humerus, when devoid of its surrounding tissues, will serve as a walking stick, hockey stick, or left-handed golf club.

The main duties of the legs are to keep the abdomen, the thorax, head and arms, off the ground and to transport them wherever they want to go. They also play a vital part in kicking, jumping, hopping and dancing, and if the knee joint is bent at a right angle, it forms either a suitable weapon for banging into somebody's face or, if placed on the ground, an adequate chair or support for the opposite sex.

The leg, as it leaves its joint with the pelvis, is divided into three main parts, namely the upper leg or thigh, which is stiffened by the femur; the lower leg between the knee joint and the foot, which is stiffened by two bones, the tibia on the inside of the leg and the fibula on the outside of the leg; and finally the foot, which is composed of a multitude of bones all in different shapes and sizes, all in different order depending on whether you walk on your toes or are flat-footed.

The thigh, or upper leg, apart from carrying the usual blood vessels, nerves, etc., down the rest of the limb, has several specialised uses of its own. It is essential for gripping cellos, motor cycle pillions, and the sides of runaway horses. In modern-day medicine, it is the favourite site for injections, and for athletes, and muscular working men, the area of choice to pull or tear a muscle, as it is quite impossible for anyone else to tell whether you have actually received an injury or not.

A cut in the back of the thigh with a sharp knife, if big enough, will ham-string the wearer and will seriously handicap him for both work and the playing of team games.

It is a practice that has tended to die out since the original Greek games and is more generally used for slowing down race-horses and greyhounds.

At the junction of the upper and lower leg is the knee joint, which is one of the most complicated joints of the body. It has a bony shield called the 'patella' on the front side of the joint (check with the nipples as to side) which to some extent shields it from frontal attacks. Similarly, you can put the knee-joint out of action by breaking the knee-cap with a hard object, such as a pneumatic drill or a footballer's boot.

Inside the joint are two pieces of gristle called 'cartilages', which are of little use other than helping Orthopaedic Surgeons to make a living by taking them out, as you can manage just as well, or even better, without them.

Cartilages have the unique property of being able to lock the knee-joint in any fixed position at any time, but it is neither the pain nor the limitation of movement of this condition that is its chief hazard. The real danger lies with medical students—and there is always one about. Even if he is only two weeks out of Grammar School and dissecting his first dogfish, he will consider he is an expert at manipulating knees, and whirls this already painful joint round and round at the slightest excuse.

Knees and lower legs are detachable and if you are unfortunate enough to fall into the hands of the keen, strong, first-year, pre-clinical medical student out to impress, this is likely to be your lot.

The knee-joints swell easily and become filled and ballooned out with fluid, similar to the soft swellings that appear on the elbows of hard drinkers. This is called either 'housemaid's knee' or 'beat knee' or even 'baggy knee', and is most socially unacceptable since it means the wearer will only be able to pull his jeans or tight trousers half way up his legs, thus limiting any anticipated evening's dancing, hop-scotch, or a long walk in the woods.

The ankle-joint, which lies between the foot and the lower leg, as well as being the common site for fractures, twists and sprains very easily. It is fortunate that the knee-cap, hovering above, points in the same direction as the toes so, in untwisting, an ankle, once again you have a landmark to guide you. It is important to keep your head in the treating of sprained ankles, because if you get your landmarks muddled up, or if by some chance the knee-cap of the limb you are treating is already behind the knee before you start untwisting the ankle, however the leg finishes up you are left with a bitter and twisted patient.

Legs come in many sizes—fat, thin, short, long, hairy, bandy. Some men walk with the knees two feet apart, others can't get one knee past the other in a single step.

Appendages To The Leg

The appendages of the leg are notable for their variety. They range from the extending hernia creeping down from the lower corners of the abdomen into the upper part of the thigh, to the huge varicose ulcer almost enclosing the ankle.

The most decorative are perhaps varicose veins that are many-coloured and swarm up the legs like snakes climbing a pillar. Alas, since free elastic stockings have been given on the National Health Service these sights of splendour have become a rarity rather than the common thing. Varicose ulcers associated with varicose veins appear all over the lower end of the leg and the wearers congregate in doctors' surgeries to compare their produce and their progress on the same lines as the local Flower Show.

At the back of the heel is the Achilles tendon which is very painful if squeezed, more painful if bitten or cut and is a favourite site for chilblains. If completely severed, like cutting the ham strings, it does tend to reduce the walking efficiency of the wearer.

The toes, which are usually between five and six in number on each foot, are of little practical use, but the gaps between the toes form creeks or harbours for the growing of athlete's foot. This is not a free pass to the Olympic Games but a type of fungus like the mushroom family and grows between the toes of most males, but is neither edible nor saleable. Toes, like the fingers can be webbed, which helps in swimming and cuts down the area for growing athlete's foot plants.

Bunions, which appear like conkers on the inside of the feet at the bottom of the big toe, are only acquired by the patient wearing winkle-picker shoes over many years. Bunions are not easy to come by. If you are not wearing the right sort of shoe to acquire them, it may mean many hours at night pulling your big toes inward manually if you are going to grow one good enough to show at the local swimming pool.

Corns—or chiropodist's delight—are pieces of hard skin found anywhere on the foot, which people who fail to acquire bunions grow, as a sort of poor man's substitute.

Feet as a whole come in many shapes and sizes like claw feet, club feet, flat feet, fat feet and the pigeon-toed species of the Chinese. They are detachable and to some extent replaceable and are important for, without them, the lower end of the lower leg tends to get worn down.

The knee-cap, already mentioned in the anatomy, is detachable, replaceable, and makes an ideal stand for a candle when detached from its surrounding tissue.

The ankle is a unit of its own. In the female it is used to attract the opposite sex. To do this, it is worn on the top of platforms, which impede walking, jam escalators, spoil polished floors, and are only useful as makeshift hammers. The habit persists, however, and it has two functions, for if the platform is high enough the wearer has to lean backwards to keep her balance, thus thrusting all her weight on to her toes, which are already kept from slipping off the platforms by a little bag at its lowest point, leaving her feet in the absolutely ideal position for bunion growing.

Anatomy of the Abdomen

The abdomen is perhaps the most variable organ in size and shape of the body components. It ranges from the slim, wasp-like structure of the male ballet dancer into the pendulous soft sack of the City Alderman. Although it has no speaking mechanism like the head and neck, it can in its own way protest audibly against both things that are done to it and put into it.

In European countries it is considered socially undesirable to communicate emotions by this method, but in the East, particuarly Arab countries, if you cannot produce at least one tummy rumble after dinner, your host will consider you have insulted his chef.

There is a way of talking, called oesophageal speech, which can be used if the vocal chords have been damaged, when wind brought up from the stomach can actually be transferred into speech.

It is difficult to outline the borders of the abdomen because, after the age of forty-five or so, the thorax or chest often slips down to merge with it. The navel, or umbilicus, is of great help in identifying it, as this is always on the abdomen. Confusion may arise, however, if this particular landmark has been removed surgically for cosmetic reasons, and an unwarily-growing hairy mole can make nonsense of all your map-reading. As a general rule, the navel, like the nipples of the thorax, show which way the wearer is moving if he is travelling in a forward direction.

The abdomen, like the thorax, contains many important organs, the main ones being the liver, spleen, kidneys, pancreas, gall bladder, stomach, and many yards of intestines, and all sorts of large veins and arteries. These structures are indispensable and although you may manage well on half one kidney or with a third of your liver, the only two that you can dispense with altogether, without any real harm, are the gall bladder and the spleen. There is a network of communication through the blood vessels in the abdomen, very similar to the outlay of Clapham Junction Goods Yard, with goods trains taking oxygen to the muscles, food from the stomach to the liver, raw materials absorbed from the intestines to factories to process it into sugar and body protein. Somewhere in the middle of the brain, in the middle of the head, there is a little office which deals with the organisation.

Protest

Indigestion, flatulence and intestinal hurry are not indications that there has been a strike in the main office, but are visible and audible protests by the stomach that it does not wish to have fourteen pints of beer, three kippers, five pickled onions, two hard-boiled eggs, five packets of potato crisps and Chinese food, all in the same evening.

Speaking on the stomach's behalf, I can say without contradiction, that there are certain things it does not like at all. These include anything that is actually on fire or burning, explosives (this does not mean laxatives), nails, glass, ironmongery, and known noxious substances such as acid, cement and liquid ammonia. Some of these tend to bung up the entrance to the food passages, while others either burn or cause holes in the side, making the whole thing leak.

The abdomen, although often the same shape and size as a punch bag, is not of the ideal material, for if pushed and prodded too hard, some of its contents may burst. Similarly, anything sharp banging on the abdomen may puncture it, letting the contents leak out. The extrusion from the abdomen of a few yards of intestine is always most inconvenient. Not only is it unsightly, but it is most difficult to get back, and this is nearly always a reason for stopping work or retiring from a game, should the circumstances arise.

Apart from the injuries to which it is susceptible, the abdomen can produce all sorts of upsets by itself. Stomach ulcers can burst, intestines can tie themselves in knots, and without the appendix to grumble, flare up and burst, half the medical profession would be on the dole.

In all these cases, the front side of the victim's abdomen (the side containing the umbilicus) becomes stiff, and the victim becomes pale and emits pain noises. The answer is not to try and destiffen the abdomen wall by kneading it with your bare feet. This will sometimes stop the victim's pain noises, but it doesn't mean he is better. It just indicates that he no longer cares.

If you want to damage a friend's kidneys, kick him in the back of the abdomen (opposite side to the umbilicus) in either right or left top corner. This is considered a most unfriendly act, because although kidneys are now replaceable, it is a tiresome business to

(a) get one to match,
(b) with the indifferent weather we have, make it grow in its new surroundings.

If, having administered your kick, your friend starts to pass blood in his water, this is an almost certain sign that you have been successful.

Kidneys and gall bladders have the ability to grow stones, and if you can put up with the pain, and it is often very painful, over the years you can acquire a matched set of balls for ear-rings from the gall bladder and a stone from the kidneys (staghorn calculus) that resembles a set of bagpipes.

The abdomen is braced at the back by part of the spine which links with the pelvis. The spine at the back of the abdomen is the favourite place to slip an intervertebral disc, which is probably the most fashionable injury known. Recovery from disc injuries is usually directly related to the date on which the wearer received compensation from whoever he is suing as being responsible for his injury. A man who has been bent double for three years, but who next day is noticed pitching hay on to a wagon, is not visible evidence of a miracle cure. It is just a sign that one more man has won his insurance claim.

The pelvis resembles two ivory water-rings joined at the front by a small bridge, called the pubis. The pelvis is attached to the spine at the back and acts like a bucket for the abdominal contents.

One leg fits into each lower corner of the pelvis, helping to keep the abdomen off the ground and thus saving it from being exposed to moulds, wet leaves, rat bites and athlete's foot.

A Portable Liquor Cask

At the lower front part of the pelvis is the bladder. This is a sort of portable elastic water carrier and has been known, when pushed, to hold up to twenty-four pints of beer.

The pelvis, when detached from the surrounding tissues, will make a good safe seat for a baby's swing, and an ideal stand for a fire extinguisher.

In the upper front part of the abdomen, between the umbilicus and the xiphisternum of the rib cage (the bit you find in the bath), is the solar plexus, and is the centre of a nerve lump, irritation of which causes interference with respiration. A sharp blow to this area, be it with a piece of scaffolding, a sledge-hammer, fist, boot, or even the point of a hockey stick, will cause the wearer to stop breathing temporarily and make various facial grimaces. It is the ideal point of contact if you want to stop somebody speaking without doing him permanent damage.

Appendages To The Abdomen

The appendages to the abdomen are interesting in that many of them are transient, i.e. they can be found one day and not the next.

This applies particularly to hernias which appear as soft lumps in the lower corners of the abdomen, called the groin. These soft lumps can vary in texture, size and colour, depending on what the wearer is doing at any particular time. If he is lying down reading the Sunday papers, all he will be able to produce is a couple of grapes, but as soon as he gets up and starts to dig the garden a couple of blood red Jaffa oranges will take their place.

Hernia-wearing is a cult. The more sophisticated carry an apparatus like crossed gun belts, called trusses, to cover them, while the less sophisticated will regale you with stories of how difficult it was pushing them back last night. The back of a truss is composed of a series of straps that look like braces, and one hernia sufferer happily wore his trusses round his shoulders for several months, well satisfied with his treatment, in spite of the fact that the vital truss pads were some feet away from the lesion they were supposed to be covering.

The sight of what looks like zip fasteners in each groin means that the wearer has at long last got fed up with wearing his gun-belt and has had his hernias surgically treated.

Hernias can grow up and around the umbilicius. It may appear to you when you see your first man with an umbilical hernia (it looks like a trunk growing out of the middle of his abdomen), that here is a man who can couple himself on to the nearest fire hydrant if he wishes to. But if you lay him on his back, most likely it will disappear.

Hernias are detachable and not replaceable, and should never be considered as possibles when searching for wrestling holds.

A Ruby's Resting Place

The other main appendage of the abdomen is the umbilicus itself, which is both detachable and replaceable, and has a myriad of uses. In the Middle East, no dancing girl is worth her salt unless she has a ruby or diamond shining from it, and now

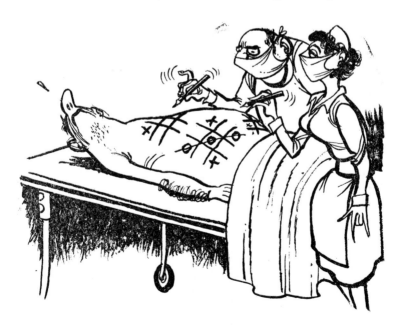

in the camping clubs of the Mediterranean they wear their name tags in them, because the rest of their wearing apparel is so brief. It must be great fun getting to know people there.

In the more sophisticated West, it is the ideal receptacle for cigarette ash after an all-night party, and is a good hiding place for micro-film, opium and your girl friend's telephone number.

The abdomen is a great site for operation scars of any sort. These will vary from thin white lines, criss-crossing over the surface, to what appears to be pieces of bacon rind interrupting the smooth surface of the skin. They have little use other than as a basis for noughts and crosses on a rainy day.

You may be confused if you see someone just after they have taken off a patterned corset or roll-on, and wonder what the hell has been going on.

CHAPTER EIGHTEEN

Off Dutyometer

SHORTLY to be released on the home market as standard equipment for practising doctors is a revolutionary piece of machinery. It has taken me some years of patient research to perfect this great contribution to medical living. It is, in simple terms, an Off Dutyometer.

It is worn round the head of practising medics and consists of a series of flashing panels of neon lights all cleverly controlled by electronics.

The panels read, in order, from the top down—

ON DUTY

OFF DUTY

ENGAGED

One switches on the panel of one's choice and then, until switched off, it will flash its message to the public at large. De luxe models are equipped with a hooter synchronised to the neon flash to emphasise further the chosen message. There is also a special adaptation for golfers, which necessitates the wearing of a second panel lower down and at the back. This gives a clear message to anyone who is approaching a doctor from behind, while he's putting, as to whether he is available for consultation or not.

The machine is also, due to its electronic construction, plus the addition of a few photoelectric cells, sensitive to certain word groups, e.g. anyone approaching the wearer of an O.

Dutyometer and saying the word group 'I know you are off duty, but . . .' will cause the machine to let out a noise like the passing of flatus and emit clouds of black smoke.

I have been conducting a personal clinical trial with the first finished model and am happy to report that since I have started to wear it I haven't had either a single unnecessary on or off duty medical request. In actual fact nobody has consulted me at all. The only real objector was the Manager of the local cinema who made me take it off when I went to see Goldfinger.

CHAPTER NINETEEN

Summing up

CLOSING this light-hearted book I would like to place on record that I consider, whatever disadvantages the National Health Service has in this country are far outweighed by its many advantages.

I believe we have the highest all-round standard of medical care in the world; I think we have the best hospitals, the best doctors, the best nurses, and even the best patients.

My confidence in the medical set-up is such that I believe it is quite big enough to stand having its leg pulled.

1974   L. PHEASANT

PS. I do not really think that British medical receptionists are hatchet-faced; in fact, I actually think they are smashing.